Rapid Antigen Testing

Edited by Laura Anfossi

Published in London, United Kingdom

Rapid Antigen Testing
http://dx.doi.org/10.5772/intechopen.104177
Edited by Laura Anfossi

Contributors
Chahinez Amira Dahmani, Ferdous Khaldi, Wassila Derouiche, Nouria Benyagoub, Lala Ghizlene Amara Zenati, Walid Hamidi, Nesserdine Bencheikh, Priya Hays, Nicole Ngai Yung Tsang, Hau Chi So, Dennis Kai Ming Ip, Marcelle Almeida Caminha, Ana Luiza Barbosa Godart Cavalcante, Rubem Figueiredo Sadok Menna-Barreto, Fariza Juliana Nordin, Lim Wan Ming, Michelle Yee Mun Teo, Lionel Lian Aun In, Natalya Rekoslavskaya, Rurik Salyaev, Alexey Stolbikov, Vanessa Susini, Chiara Sanguinetti, Silvia Ursino, Laura Caponi, Maria Franzini, Andrés Álvarez-Rodríguez, Magdalena Radwanska, Stefan Magez, Steven Odongo

First published in London, United Kingdom, 2023 by IntechOpen
IntechOpen is the global imprint of INTECHOPEN LIMITED, registered in England and Wales, registration number: 11086078, 5 Princes Gate Court, London, SW7 2QJ, United Kingdom

British Library Cataloguing-in-Publication Data
A catalogue record for this book is available from the British Library

Additional hard and PDF copies can be obtained from orders@intechopen.com

Rapid Antigen Testing
Edited by Laura Anfossi
p. cm.
Print ISBN 978-1-83769-568-3
Online ISBN 978-1-83769-567-6
eBook (PDF) ISBN 978-1-83769-569-0

Meet the editor

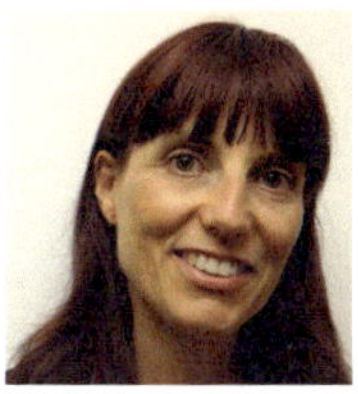

Laura Anfossi received an MS in Chemistry and a Ph.D. in Biochemical Sciences from the University of Torino, Italy, in 1997 and 2001, respectively. She has been a Full Professor of Analytical Chemistry at the Department of Chemistry, University of Torino Since 2022. Her main research interest is the development of innovative immunodiagnostic methods and immunosensors based on natural antibodies and synthetic ligands, such as molecularly imprinted polymers and aptamers. She has participated in and led several research projects and co-authored more than 140 peer-reviewed papers and 6 book chapters.

Contents

Preface

Rapid antigen tests generally refer to analytical devices for detecting macromolecular biomarkers by using the lateral flow assay (LFA) technique. This analytical system typically comes in the form of strips made of porous cellulosic materials that enable the establishment of a capillary flow when put into contact with a liquid sample. Along the strip, reactive zones are created by sticking selective recognition elements (such as antibodies, nucleic acids, receptors, etc.). In addition, the device also includes a signal reporter, which is responsible for the generation of the signal. Common signal reporters include colored/fluorescent nano or microparticles so that the signal is detected by the unaided eye or through portable optical readers. Although other detection strategies have been proposed, for example, the incorporation of Raman tags linked to metal nanoparticles to enable surface-enhanced Raman spectroscopy (SERS) detection [1, 2], commercial devices currently rely only on the use of colorimetric and fluorescent detection [3, 4].

LFAs are defined as LFIAs (lateral flow immunoassays) when the selective recognition elements are represented by specific antibodies, and NALFIAs (nucleic acid lateral flow assays) when specificity is achieved through the complementarity between nucleic acid sequences. In this second category, aptamers deserve a separate discussion, as they are oligonucleotide sequences; however, they are able to bind to various molecules of different chemical nature, beyond hybridizing with complementary strands.

Antigen detection is accomplished by dropping the liquid sample, eventually containing the antigen, at one end of the device (or dipping the terminal part of the device directly into the liquid sample). The liquid flows through the porous membranes and, during the route towards the other end of the strip, first comes into contact with the detector (labelled selective) and then encounters one or more reactive zones made of immobilized recognition elements, usually in the form of lines perpendicular to the flow direction. If any antigen molecules are present in the sample, they react with the detector and are captured by the bioligands in the reactive zone so that the result is the accumulation of the detector in the reactive zone, where the antigen acts as a bridge between the two. The reactive zone sensitive to the presence of the antigen is usually referred to as the "test line." A second reactive zone is commonly added, which is called the "control line," to indicate that the device is working properly and to assure the reliability of the test line response. The control line is composed of a second bioligand, which can capture the detector regardless of the presence of the antigen. Therefore, the appearance of a detectable signal at the test line confirms the existence of the antigen in the sample (at a level above the detection limit of the assay), while the signal at the control line represents the correct functioning of the device. Typically, two colored (fluorescent) lines are indicative of a positive sample, while negative samples generate a signal only at the control line.

The distinctive features of the LFA platform that contribute to its clinical success, especially as a tool for diagnosing infectious diseases, are summarized in the ASSURED criteria [5]: Affordability, Sensitivity, Specificity, User-friendliness, Rapidity, Equipment-freeness, and Deliverability. Meeting all these requirements allows for the practical use of LFA as a point-of-care test or near-patient test as well as for home/self-testing.

This kind of test has become enormously popular due to the COVID-19 pandemic. The tremendous demand for timely deliverable and cost-effective analytical tools to cope with the billions of tests required during pandemic waves highlights the role that rapid antigen tests can play in the management of infectious disease outbreaks. However, the use of these diagnostic tools has been questioned and their practical utility is still controversial, mostly because of concerns raised about their performance in comparison with molecular techniques.

This book provides a comprehensive overview of rapid antigen testing. Chapters 1 and 2 compare the analytical and diagnostic performance of rapid testing with other diagnostic approaches such as molecular testing. The chapters review and discuss the benefits and limitations of the various strategies.

Along with showing that the diagnostic merits of rapid antigen diagnostic (RAD) tests fit with requirements for accurate identification of infected subjects, the chapters clearly identify some peculiar characteristics of rapid antigen tests that rendered them especially useful in the context of the pandemic. The reduced costs and simplicity of RAD tests (which overcome the need for trained personnel) enabled their massive and diffuse use, even in those countries where access to care is limited. Chapter 3 discusses the affordability of these tests as a turning point in the worldwide fight against COVID-19. The same benefit has been recognized as an opportunity to counteract other infectious diseases, as discussed in Chapter 4, especially in developing countries where the limitation of funds and the lack of infrastructures and trained personnel often prevent the application of efficient strategies to limit the transmission of infections.

The pandemic has prompted the search for new and improved assay formats to meet the requirement of high sensitivity. Moreover, the identification of alternative biorecognition elements to replace antibodies has been largely pursued. Chapter 5 discusses the development of aptamers as a promising strategy to prepare in vitro bioligands with high affinity and specificity, comparable to those of natural antibodies as also discussed in Chapter 6. As selective ligands, aptamers have been used successfully to develop rapid tests, keeping the same advantages of antibody-based approaches while meeting the requirements of the 3Rs principles of the National Centre for the Replacement, Refinement & Reduction of Animals in Research [6].

Chapters 7 and 8 address the continuous improvement of immunoassay performance through using high-affinity bioligands.

In summary, the popularity of RAD tests as convenient diagnostic tools to supplement other well-established strategies for detecting protein biomarkers in biological fluids, together with the limitations recognized in their performance, represent an open challenge for research to optimize existing approaches (which can still largely be improved), suggesting new system design, replacing natural antibodies by innovative bioligands. However, the benefit of the practical application of point-of-care and near-patient testing can no longer be underestimated.

Laura Anfossi
Department of Chemistry,
University of Torino,
Turin, Italy

References

[1] Yadav S, Sadique MA, Ranjan P, Kumar N, Singhal A, Srivastava AK, et al. SERS based lateral flow immunoassay for point-of-care detection of SARS-CoV-2 in clinical samples. ACS Applied Bio Materials. 2021;**4**:2974-2995. DOI: 10.1021/acsabm.1c00102

[2] Sloan-Dennison S, O'Connor E, Dear JW, Graham D, Faulds K. Towards quantitative point of care detection using SERS lateral flow immunoassays. Analytical and Bioanalytical Chemistry. 2022;**414**:4541-4549. DOI: 10.1007/s00216-022-03933-8

[3] Park J. Lateral flow immunoassay reader technologies for quantitative point-of-care testing. Sensors. 2022;**22**:7398. DOI: 10.3390/s22197398

[4] Di Nardo F, Chiarello M, Cavalera S, Baggiani C, Anfossi L. Ten years of lateral flow immunoassay technique applications: Trends, challenges and future perspectives. Sensors. 2021;**21**:5185. DOI: 10.3390/s21155185

[5] Otoo JA, Schlappi TS. REASSURED multiplex diagnostics: A critical review and forecast. Biosensors (Basel). 2022;**12**(2):124. DOI: 10.3390/bios12020124

[6] Animals in science. EU actions for the protection of animals used for scientific purposes. Available from: https://environment.ec.europa.eu/topics/chemicals/animals-science_en#:~:text=EU%20legislation%20on%20animals%20in,which%20first%20appeared%20in%201959%20

Section 1

Rapid Tests for Communicable Diseases

Chapter 1

Comparison between RT-qPCR and LAMP Methods for a Rapid COVID-19 Diagnosis in an Algerian Sample

Chahinez Amira Dahmani, Ferdous Khaldi, Wassila Derouiche, Nouria Benyagoub, Lala Ghizlene Amara Zenati, Walid Hamidi and Nesserdine Bencheikh

Abstract

Accurate and rapid diagnostic tests are critical for achieving control of COVID-19, a pandemic illness caused by severe acute respiratory syndrome coronavirus-2 (SARS-CoV-2). Diagnostic tests for COVID-19 fall into two main categories: molecular and antigen tests. The reverse transcription real-time-quantitative polymerase chain reaction (RT-qPCR) has become the gold standard for diagnosis of the COVID-19; however, this test has many limitations that include potential false-negative results and precarious availability of test materials. The isothermal PCR or Loop-Mediated Isothermal Amplification (LAMP) method has generated substantial interest as an alternative or complement to RT-qPCR, as some might be cheaper and easier to implement at the point of care. To our knowledge, it is the first Algerian study that wanted to compare two different molecular biology methods: RT-qPCR and LAMP for rapid diagnosis of COVID-19. In this review, we wanted to compare the CTs observed by RT-qPCR with those observed by LAMP in the same laboratory.

Keywords: COVID-19, SARS-Cov-2, RT-qPCR, LAMP, threshold CT

1. Introduction

The large-scale transmission of viral diseases poses a serious threat to global public health. In recent decades, several viral epidemics have emerged with increasing frequency, including severe acute respiratory syndrome coronavirus (SARS-CoV) and, more recently, Middle East respiratory syndrome coronavirus (MERS-CoV). Recently, a novel coronavirus (SARS-CoV-2) emerged in Wuhan province in China. Therefore, a global pandemic affected the working and living conditions of billions of people worldwide in late December 2019, in Wuhan. It is known as COVID-19 (Coronavirus Disease 2019), and this novel coronavirus rapidly spreads through China and then many other countries globally. Consequently, the World Health

Organization (WHO) has declared COVID-19 an international public health emergency and has given a very high-risk assessment on a global level.

The COVID-19 disease has clinical manifestations that highly vary from individual to individual, ranging from mild flu-like symptoms to sometimes life-threatening conditions. Hence, the accurate diagnosis of COVID-19 is challenging. Routine clinical diagnosis of this outbreak is confirmed by several laboratory detection methods, including nucleic acid amplification tests and serological techniques. However, in some patients, the transit of immunity is delayed due to individual risk factors such as older age and co-morbidities like diabetes, hypertension, cardiopathy, and obesity [1, 2].

The SARS-CoV-2 virus testing and corresponding human antibodies are essential for the COVID-19 diagnosis and treatment. It is important to underline that this screening was also considered a prerequisite for different economic and social activities such as international flights, offline work, access to shopping malls as well as sporting and social events. For this, an unimaginable number of rapid molecular tests for COVID-19 have been carried out in numerous medical institutions.

It is evident that the reverse transcription real-time-quantitative polymerase chain reaction (RT-qPCR) still remains a gold standard in the detection of the coronavirus, but an immediate need for alternative less expensive, more rapid tests is clear. As for COVID-19 testing, the majority of countries have performed many RT-qPCR tests per 1000 people by now. This puts an additional constraint on the country's economy. RT-qPCR tests that constitute the predominant part of these numbers cost on average DA2000–5000 (£20–50) per test. Not to mention the costs of electricity, equipment maintenance, and salaries for staff. For this reason, some laboratories have considered adopting new techniques such as LAMP (Loop-Mediated Isothermal Amplification).

Precisely, several studies published in 2021 have suggested that RT-LAMP seems to be a diagnostic tool for COVID-19 as an alternative to RT-qPCR, especially in the acute symptomatic phase of COVID-19 [3, 4]. Then in 2022, a meta-analysis carried out on 19 studies showed that the LAMP method is faster and highly specific for the detection of SARS-CoV-2 compared to RT-qPCR [5].

In Algeria, the SARS-Cov-2 RT-qPCR test is available at the COVID-19 services of various hospitals, some university laboratories, and at all Algerian Pasteur Institutes. In addition, some Algerian COVID-19 services have adopted the LAMP technique, such as the COVID-19 Laboratory of the University of Mostaganem, Algeria. You should also know that the results of an RT-PCR or RT-LAMP test can be reported in viral load (CV) (x copies/ml) or in threshold cycle value (Ct) between 0 and 40. The values Ct are inversely correlated with CV and the correlation formula varies according to the diagnostic platform used. The aim of this study was first to compare the CTs found using the different RT-qPCR kits at the COVID-19 laboratory of the University of Mostaganem. Furthermore, we wanted to compare the CTs observed by RT-qPCR with those observed by LAMP in the same laboratory. To our knowledge, this is the first study that tries to compare these two important molecular techniques for the diagnosis of COVID-19 in Algeria.

2. Comparison test between RT-qPCR and LAMP in COVID-19 diagnosis

Coronavirus is a positive-sense single-stranded RNA virus. The viral envelope consists of a lipid bilayer where the membrane (M), envelope (E), and spike (S) structural proteins are anchored. A subset of coronaviruses (in particular, beta coronavirus) also have a shorter spike-like surface protein called hemagglutinin esterase

(HE). Inside the envelope, there is the nucleocapsid, which is formed from multiple copies of the nucleocapsid (N) protein. This protein is bound to the single-stranded RNA genome. The lipid bilayer envelope, membrane proteins, and nucleocapsid protect the virus when it is outside the host cell [6–13].

Some World Centers for Disease Control and Prevention rapidly employed molecular assays for the detection of COVID-19, mostly, employing the development of real-time polymerase chain reaction (RT-PCR) methods to diagnose COVID-19 [1]. Molecular tests for the SARS-Cov2 virus use improved quantitative RT-PCR methods characterized by rapid detection, high sensitivity, and specificity. These tests target various genetic combinations according to the already published protein and genomic structure of this virus. The genes mainly targeted are Open Reading Frame (ORF) gene, envelope (E) gene, nucleocapsid (N), and RNA-dependent RNA polymerase (RdRp) gene [14–19]. However, other new PCR-based methods like the LAMP (Loop-Mediated Isothermal Amplification) method also show higher and improved specificity and test sensitivity.

2.1 The reverse transcription real-time PCR (RT-qPCR)

RT-qPCR is a technique that makes it possible to perform quantitative PCR from an RNA sample. RNA is first reverse transcribed using an enzyme called reverse transcriptase, which allows the synthesis of complementary DNA (cDNA). As in conventional PCR, the cycles of a conventional quantitative PCR reaction can take place in three steps: denaturation, hybridization, and elongation. However, in RT-qPCR, fluorescent labeling allows data collection as the PCR progresses, and it can be done in one or two steps. "One step" tests combine reverse transcription and PCR in a single tube and buffer. Regarding "two-step" RT-qPCR, reverse transcription and PCR are performed in separate tubes, with different optimized buffers.

To reduce the risk of false positives from the amplification of any contaminating genomic DNA, it is best to design primers for the qPCR step of RT-qPCR at a region that spans an exon-exon junction.

Ideally, all RT-qPCR experiments should include a negative reverse transcription control (−RT control) to test for contaminating DNA. Of course, like any PCR reaction, this control contains all of the reaction components except the reverse transcriptase. Therefore, if PCR amplification is observed, it is most likely derived from the contaminating DNA [20, 21].

2.2 The LAMP (loop-mediated isothermal amplification)

Loop-Mediated Isothermal Amplification (LAMP) is a novel isothermal nucleic acid amplification method. The classic PCR has been used for pathogen detection for more than 30 years. The process of this new technique uses high temperatures to denature the DNA, then the temperatures are cooled, and the primers bind to the DNA. Thus, to detect pathogens such as SARS-Cov-2, it is sufficient to program repeated cycles of high and low temperatures and primers for DNA amplification.

Unlike conventional PCR, LAMP uses four to six primers to recognize six distinct regions of DNA or RNA. LAMP primers cause displacement of the DNA strand and cause a loop to form at the end of the DNA strand. This structure allows the exponential accumulation of additional double-stranded DNA and is the basis for amplification [21].

Numerous studies have now shown the successful application of LAMP assays in various forms to detect coronavirus RNA in patient samples, demonstrating that 1–10 copies of viral RNA template per reaction were sufficient for successful detection, which were ~ 100-fold more sensitive than conventional RT-PCR methods [22–28]. The LAMP method does not contain a double-stranded DNA purification or denaturation step, which explains the speed of the analysis.

LAMP is currently one of the most widely used isothermal methods, and it has quickly taken its place in molecular biology laboratories, especially those that do not have PCR equipment. It is a simple and rapid DNA/RNA amplification method that takes place in a thermocycler or a water bath at 65°C. It was developed by *Notomi et al,* in 2000 and developed by the Japanese company Eiken Chemical Company (Tokyo) [29]. LAMP also uses bioluminescence to detect the pathogen where target amplification takes only 15 minutes. However, as with any emerging technology, LAMP has some drawbacks. For example, it presents a risk of contamination by other nucleic acids, and it does not allow the amplification of fragments that exceed 300 base pairs (bp). Another disadvantage is the perceived complexity of the methodology, requiring a complex primer design system that may limit selection and resolution or target site specificity.

3. Comparison study between the kits used for the rapid diagnosis of COVID-19 in algeria

Importantly, different RT-qPCR protocols use different primer-probe sets targeting various segments of the SARS-CoV-2 genome. These protocols may not have the same analytical or clinical sensitivity and specificity, even when used for the same COVID-19 sample [30]. It should also be noted that different RT-qPCR kits designed for the detection of SARS-CoV-2 have different reagents. A recent study comparing the contents of four kits developed by different institutions (US CDC, China CDC, Germany CU, and the University of Hong Kong) showed that even when the tests are identical, their concentrations in the reaction mixture can be different [31–33]. Some researchers critically compared the analytical efficiencies and sensitivities of these four RT-qPCR assays, and each of them is likely to have different sensitivity/specificity, and possibly different accuracies. They concluded that all the primer-probe sets for these four assays can be used to detect SARSCoV-2 as long as the limitations of each assay are recognized (DANAFORM®). However, they noted that the different assays are capable to differentiate between true negatives and positives when a low load of SARS-CoV-2 is present in a given sample [34].

3.1 Study design

This is a retrospective study carried out at the level of the molecular biology laboratory of Mostaganem from January 01, 2021, to December 01, 2022.

Out of a total of 7021 samples received at our laboratory, only 6595 were retained. In our study, the samples were taken either in hospitals or in the universities of the province of Mostaganem. The exclusion criteria were noncompliant samples, incomplete information sheets, and inconclusive tests.

Viral RNA extraction was performed from the swab samples immediately in the COVID-19 laboratory of Mostaganem using the RNeasy Micro Kit (QIAGEN, GERMANY).

The samples were treated with nine different RT-qPCR kits: QuantiNova COVID-19-Imd, Da An Gene, Gene Proof, Sansure Biotech, Allplex, Cosaryon One Stepimd-, Thaiduong, and Snibe. The RT-qPCR was performed according to the protocols defined in respective technical sheets for each kit on two thermocyclers available in our laboratory (Bioer Line Gene Mini and QIAGEN Rotor-Gene Q).

DOI: http://dx.doi.org/10.5772/intechopen.1001116

In addition, the nasopharyngeal swab samples obtained from 33 COVID-19 patients were tested by RT-LAMP and that were already genotyped by RT-qPCR before. We started the study in January 2022 and unfortunately stopped when the reagents ran out.

Sensitivities and specificities of RT-LAMP compared with RT-qPCR were analyzed as a function of the CT values. The goal was to observe if there would be a noticeable difference between the results of the two methods.

For that, we used the "Smart Amp™ 2019 New Coronavirus Detection Reagent" co-developed by DNAFORM Corporation (Yokohama, Japan) and RIKEN (Yokohama, Japan) for LAMP. We also compared the RT-qPCR kits used for these 33 samples. These kits are QuantiNova COVID-19-Imd, Gene Proof, and Sansure Biotech. Afterward, we compared these three RT-qPCR kits with the LAMP Smart Amp kit.

3.1.1 QuantiNova kit (Germany)

The QuantiNova Multiplex RT-PCR Kit is intended for molecular biology applications. This product is not intended for the diagnosis, prevention, or treatment of a disease.

3.1.2 Sansure Biotech kit (China)

SARS-CoV-2 and Influenza A/B Virus Multiplex Nucleic Acid Diagnostic Kit (PCR-Fluorescence Probing) (PCR-Fluorescence Probing). It is used for the detection of SARS-CoV-2 for two RdRp targets (IP2 and IP4).

3.1.3 Gene Proof SARS-CoV-2 PCR Kit (Czech)

The kit has been manufactured according to Directive 98/79/EC of the European Parliament as an in vitro diagnostic medical device and has been designed for professional use in clinical and specialized research laboratories. It detects the specific sequences of the virus genome (RdRp gene, E gene, and N gene) in a single reaction. The multiplex targeting mechanism ensures high sensitivity of SARS-CoV-2 detection.

3.1.4 Smart Amp SARS-CoV-2 Test (Russia)

The EMG Smart Amp SARS-Cov-2 RNA Detection kit is designed to detect the viral material presence in biological samples by implementing reverse transcription and real-time isothermal amplification reactions. It is characterized by a Fast Reaction Rate Typically 10 minutes–35 minutes, High Sensitivity From 100 copies, and High Specificity. It detects and identifies four target genes for SARS-CoV-2 using multiplex real-time PCR SARS-CoV-2 Assay.

3.2 RT-qPCR and RT-LAMP comparison

We have presented all the characteristics of the different kits used in the COVID-19 laboratory of the University of Mostaganem (**Table 1**).

As shown in **Table 1**, all RT-qPCR kits are composed of probes that detect a maximum of two different genes of the Sars-Cov2 virus (detection channels: FAM, ROX/TEXAS RED, CYS, and/or JOE/VIC) except the Gene Proof kit which targets three genes with a single common probe (FAM). However, the Smart Amp Kit is an RT-LAMP assay that can perform both reverse transcriptase and isothermal DNA amplification reactions in a single reaction tube (**Table 1**). We have also mentioned the duration determined for each RT-qPCR or RT-LAMP kit.

Also, we have provided an evaluation of our RT-qPCR and RT-LAMP tests with their different indicators of positivity, i.e., cycle threshold values (Ct). Indeed, knowledge of diagnostic tests for COVID-19 highlights the need for local validation of positive–negative Ct cutoff values when establishing RT-qPCR assays for the detection of SARS-CoV-2.

The threshold cycle value (Ct) is the actual number of cycles required for the PCR to detect the virus. It gives an estimate of the likely amount of virus present in the original sample. If the virus was found in a small number of cycles (Ct value less than 35), it means that it was easy to find in the sample, and therefore the sample contained a large amount of it.

3.3 Statistical analysis

The Pearson's Chi-square test (2x2 table) for data analysis was used for numerous parameters such as sensitivity, specificity, negative and positive tests, and CT values. A P value <0.05 was considered statistically significant.

Summary statistics in **Tables 2** and **3** are presented as the mean and standard error of the mean. All statistical analyses were performed with SPSS (IBM.SPSS. v.22.).

RT-PCR Kits	Reading channels				Time	CT values
	FAM	ROX/TEXAS RED	CYS	JOE/VIC		
IMD	RdRp	Nsp9	/	IC	123 min	35
SANSURE	ORF	N	IC	/	118 min	40
Cosaryon	N	/	/	IC	76 min	40
GenePROOF	RdRp/E/N	/	/	IC	120 min	35
Da An gene	N	/	IC	ORF	132 min	40
Thaiduong	N3	N1	IC	N2	149 min	40
Snibe	ORF	N	/	IC	87 min	40
Allplex	/	/	IC	RdRp	106 min	35
QuantiNova	RdRp	Nsp9	/	IC	120 min	35
Smart Amp	Smart cible	/	/	/	45 min	35

FAM, ROX, CYS, JOE/VIC: reading qPCR channels. Open Reading Frame: ORF gene, Envelope: E gene, Nucleocapsid: N gene, the Non-structural protein 9: Nsp9 gene, and RNA-dependent RNA polymerase: RdRp gene. CI: Internal Control, min: minute, CT values: Cycle Threshold.

Table 1.
The targeted genes by the different channels for each kit used in the Mostaganem COVID-19 laboratory.

	RT-qPCR (n = 33)	LAMP (n = 33)
CT mean ± SE	25.55 ± 7.14	23.04 ± 8.82
P value	0.23	

N: number, CT: cycle threshold, SE: Standard Error. P-value <0.05 is statically significant.

Table 2.
Comparison between all samples treated by the RT-qPCR kits with the LAMP kit.

RT-PCR kits/Smart Amp kit	Mean CT	Standard Deviation	P value
QuantiNova (n = 18)	26.50	4.87	0.24
vs. *Smart Amp (n = 18)*	18.86	9.52	
Sansure (n = 04)	37.01	3.95	0.26
vs. *Smart Amp (n = 04)*	31.18	0.93	
Gene Proof (n = 12)	20.64	6.12	0.23
vs. *Smart Amp (n = 12)*	27.22	4.39	

N: number of samples. CT: cycle threshold. SD: Standard Deviation. P value <0.05 is statically significant.

Table 3.
Comparison between the 33 samples treated by the three RT-qPCR kits with the LAMP kit.

The graphical tables and histograms were designed by Microsoft Excel Software (for Windows.11).

3.4 Ethic statement

The study was approved by the Institutional Review Board of the University of Mostaganem.

4. Results

RT-qPCR and RT-LAMP kits characteristics:

All the kits used in our laboratory are kept at −20 C ° except the Cosaryon One Step-IMD kit (kept at room temperature) and the Snibe kit (2 and 8°C) before its reconstruction.

Since the outbreak of the COVID-19 pandemic in 2020, we have observed that the Gene Proof kit has been used the most in our laboratory. But this is due only to the high availability of the latter.

As shown in **Table 1**, the Smart AMP kit is the only one that uses isothermal PCR, and suddenly it is the fastest test (45 minutes). In addition, concerning the RT-qPCR, the Thai Duong kit is the slowest test (149 minutes), while the Cosaryon test is the fastest (76 minutes).

Hoffmann's meta-analysis also found a time variation ranging from 30 to 60 minutes, which in any case makes RT-LAMP an extremely fast method compared to RT-PCR, which requires about 120 to 160 min to complete [5].

The Ct value is influenced by several factors, including the PCR test kit used, the time of sample collection, the machine used for analysis, the technique used by the healthcare professional to obtain the sample, and the sample type (collection method). In our present work, CT threshold values were determined according to the validation methods of the COVID-19 laboratory in Mostaganem for each kit. Indeed, some RT-qPCR kits have a CT threshold = 35 and others = 40; however, the RT-LAMP (Smart Amp) kit has a CT threshold determined of 35 (**Table 1**).

Several studies have analyzed the effect of the CT threshold value on the diagnosis of COVID-19. Mainly, the study by Serrano-Cumplido et al. in 2021 [35] summarized the different possibilities of CT values obtained during an RT-qPCR reaction. The study was carried out on a sample of the Spanish population and concluded that CT values <30 determine an acute COVID-19 infection, CT values between 30 and 34 determine a moderate infection, and CT values between 34 and 37 are considered undetermined values. Finally, CT values >37 would rather indicate the absence of the SARS-Cov-2 virus. These threshold values can be slightly modified from one laboratory to another and according to the molecular kits used [35].

It should also be noted that all the kits used in this study target a maximum of two different genes (ORF gene, N gene, Nsp9 gene, and/or RdRp gene) except the Gene Proof kit target three different SARS-CoV-2 genes (RdRp gene, E gene, and N gene) at the same time with a common probe (FAM) (**Table 1**).

RT-qPCR and RT-LAMP kits comparison:

Otherwise, to achieve our goal of comparing the RT-qPCR and LAMP methods in the detection of the SARS-Cov-2 virus, we succeeded in comparing 33 samples determined by three RT-qPCR kits (QuantiNova, Sansure, and Gene Proof) with the Smart Amp kit of the LAMP method.

As shown in **Table 2**, we have observed that the mean of the CT thresholds obtained by the LAMP method of the 33 samples is lower than that obtained by the RT-qPCR. This difference was not statically significant ($p > 0.05$) (**Table 2**).

As shown in **Table 3**, we compared each sample determined separately by an RT-qPCR kit with the RT-LAMP (Smart Amp) kit. Again, we found no statistically significant difference between mean CT ($p > 0.05$).

Furthermore, we have noted that there is a strong difference in the average CTs between the kits. Indeed, the average CT between the two kits QuantiNova and Sansure is much higher than that obtained by LAMP (respectively 26.50 vs. 18.86 and 37.01 vs. 31.18). However, the average CT obtained by the Gene Proof kit is rather lower than that of Smart Amp (20.64 vs. 27.22, respectively).

The study by Inaba M et al. analyzed the sensitivity and specificity of the LAMP method compared to RT-qPCR. Inaba's team showed that the sensitivity and

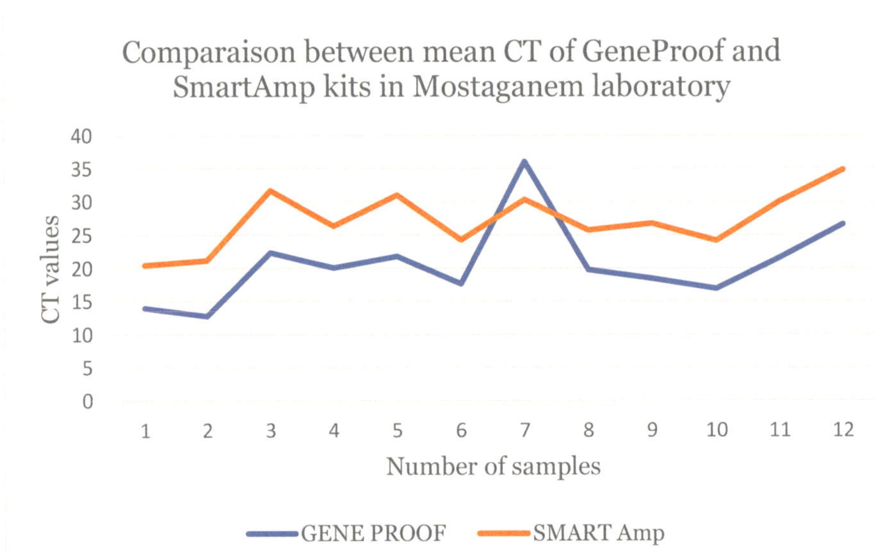

Figure 1.
Line chart which shows the difference between the CT values obtained by the Gene Proof kit (RT-qPCR) and those obtained by the Smart Amp kit (LAMP).

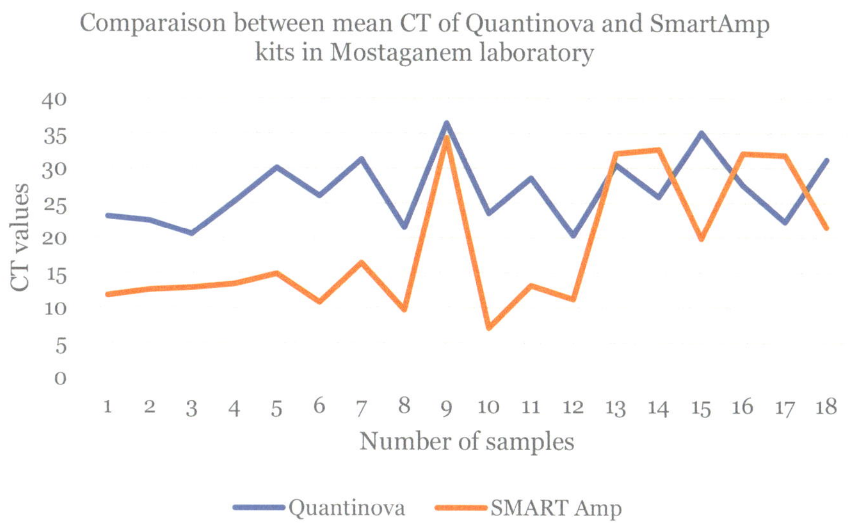

Figure 2.
Line chart which shows the difference between the CT values obtained by the QuantiNova kit (RT-qPCR) and those obtained by the Smart Amp kit (LAMP).

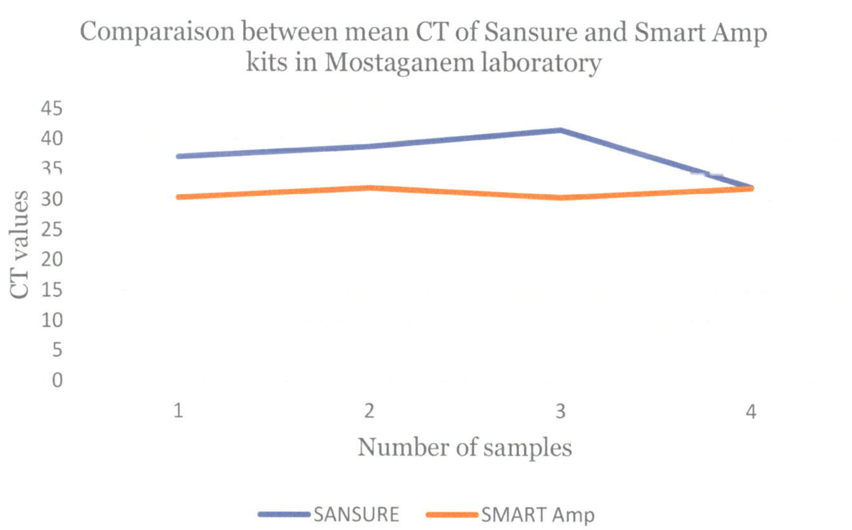

Figure 3.
Line chart which shows the difference between the CT values obtained by the Sansure kit (RT-qPCR) and those obtained by the Smart Amp kit (LAMP).

specificity of RT-LAMP were 100%. This suggests that the LAMP method has the same reliability as RT-qPCR [3].

On the other hand, the following figures demonstrate and confirm these observations regarding the use of the two COVID-19 detection techniques in Algeria (**Figures 1–3**).

According to **Figure 1**, we can confirm that the CT values obtained by the Gene Proof kit (Blue line) are better than the CT values obtained by the Smart Amp kit (Orange line). Also, only one sample found to be COVID-19 negative (CT = 36.02) by RT-qPCR was found COVID-19 positive (CT = 30.32) by the LAMP.

Figures 2 and **3** show the difference between the CT values obtained by the two RT-qPCR kits and those obtained by isothermal PCR. It is clear that the orange lines are lower than the blue lines (**Figure 2** and **3**). This once again confirms the effectiveness of the LAMP method in the detection of the SARS-Cov-2 virus. Moreover, several negative COVID-19 cases by the RT-qPCR kits (QuantiNova and Sansure) were found to be rather COVID-19 positive by the LAMP Smart Amp kit. This suggests that the LAMP method can identify individuals determined to be "COVID-19 negative" by RT-qPCR as "false negatives".

Although the Ct value does not indicate the severity of the disease, it could play an important role in clinical and public health decision-making if carefully analyzed along with other factors such as the type of test used, the history of exposure to COVID-19, symptoms, and individual patient characteristics. This analysis is done by health professionals and laboratories, who fully understand all the factors under study [35].

The efficiency of the LAMP is logical given the detection principle developed for this method using a set of six primers that target eight regions of SARS-Cov-2. In addition, the Gene Proof kit also has the ability to target three SARS-Cov-2 genes using a common probe, and this explains the results obtained by comparing it with the LAMP Smart Amp kit. We concluded that the LAMP with its many advantages (speed, simplicity, etc.) can replace RT-qPCR in the search for SARS-Cov-2, especially when the kits on the market are not adapted to a given ethnic population.

5. Conclusion

It cannot be denied that the RT-qPCR diagnostic assays used have high sensitivity and specificity, making them the gold standard for COVID-19 diagnosis. In addition, it must be emphasized that the different kits developed for the RT-qPCR method to detect SARS-Cov-2 use different sets of primer probes targeting various segments of the SARS-CoV-2 genome.

These kits/tests have different sensitivity/specificity and possibly different accuracies. However, it is a lengthy method and requires complex equipment and a highly skilled operator. In order to safely return to normal life, a test needs to be rapid, portable, and have enough analytical sensitivity to maintain a 90% or higher true positive rate. Loop-Mediated Isothermal Amplification (LAMP) is a method of nucleic acid amplification that exhibits increased sensitivity and specificity that are significantly rapid and do not require expensive reagents or instruments, which aids in cost reduction for coronavirus detection.

Since the start of the pandemic, the real-time RT-qPCR test has been the gold standard for diagnosing SARS-CoV-2. Unfortunately, cases of false negatives have also been reported due to different issues: sample collection, sample transport, and viral RNA extraction. Indeed, RT-qPCR assays have many limitations such as a high workload that requires skilled operators for testing and sample collection as well as expensive instruments and well-equipped laboratories.

In this study, we wanted to compare these two molecular biology methods capable of detecting SARS-Cov-2 in Algeria. Indeed, we amplified the same sample taken at random from the COVID-19 laboratory in Mostaganem (already determined by RT-qPCR) by isothermal PCR (LAMP) using the Smart Amp kit. Even though our sample size is not large, LAMP is an ultrasensitive nucleic acid amplification method that can detect minute quantities of DNA or RNA templates within roughly an hour, far outstripping normally utilized RT-PCR methods, particularly with the current demands for rapid and sensitive testing.

This original study is only an initial part of a long work that remains to be done by our team at the University of Mostaganem. It would be interesting to increase the size of the sample and that other laboratories also get involved.

Acknowledgements

We would like to thank **Professor Nesserdine BENCHIKH**, director of the COVID-19 molecular laboratory at the University of Mostaganem for giving us access to the various information required for the development of this work. We also thank **Mr. Mehdi DAHMANI** for his precious help concerning the statistical part of this study.

Conflict of interest

The authors declare no conflict of interest.

Author details

Chahinez Amira Dahmani[1*], Ferdous Khaldi[2], Wassila Derouiche[1,2], Nouria Benyagoub[1,2], Lala Ghizlene Amara Zenati[1,2], Walid Hamidi[1,2] and Nesserdine Bencheikh[1,2]

1 University of Mostaganem "Abdelhamid Ibn Badis", Algeria

2 University Hospital Center of Mostaganem, Algeria

*Address all correspondence to: chahinezamira.dahmani@univ-mosta.dz

References

[1] Corman VM, Landt O, Kaiser M, Molenkamp R, Meijer A, Chu DK, et al. Detection of 2019 novel coronavirus (2019-nCoV) by real-time RT-PCR. European Communicable Disease Bulletin. 2020;**25**:30 Epub 2020/01/30

[2] Wan Y, Shang J, Graham R, Baric RS, Li F. Receptor Recognition by the Novel Coronavirus from Wuhan: An analysis based on decade-long structural studies of SARS coronavirus. Journal of Virology. 2020;**94**:7 Epub 2020/01/31

[3] Inaba M, Higashimoto Y, Toyama Y, Horiguchi T, Hibino M, Iwata M, et al. Diagnostic accuracy of LAMP versus PCR over the course of SARS-CoV-2 infection. International Journal of Infectious Diseases: IJID: Official publication of the International Society for Infectious Diseases. 2021;**107**:195-200 Epub 2021/04/17

[4] Baba MM, Bitew M, Fokam J, Lelo EA, Ahidjo A, Asmamaw K, et al. Diagnostic performance of a colorimetric RT-LAMP for the identification of SARS-CoV-2: A multicenter prospective clinical evaluation in sub-Saharan Africa. EClinicalMedicine. 2021;**40**:101101 Epub 2021/09/04

[5] da Rosa E, Hoffmann TMD, Ghiotto MA, Gaboardi G, Cantarelli VV. Performance of loop-mediated isothermal amplification (LAMP) targeting the Nucleocapsid (N) gene of SARS-CoV-2 for rapid diagnosis of COVID-19. Systematic Review and Meta-Analysis. COVID. 2022;**2**:759-766

[6] Belouzard S, Chu VC, Whittaker GR. Activation of the SARS coronavirus spike protein via sequential proteolytic cleavage at two distinct sites. Proceedings of the National Academy of Sciences of the United States of America. 2009;**106**(14):5871-5876 Epub 2009/03/27

[7] Bosch BJ, van der Zee R, de Haan CA, Rottier PJ. The coronavirus spike protein is a class I virus fusion protein: Structural and functional characterization of the fusion core complex. Journal of Virology. 2003;**77**(16):8801-8811 Epub 2003/07/30

[8] Alic S, Dermastia M, Burger J, Dickinson M, Pietersen G, Dreo T. Genome-informed design of a LAMP assay for the specific detection of the strain of 'Candidatus Phytoplasma asteris' Phytoplasma occurring in grapevines in South Africa. Plant Disease. 2022;**106**(11):2927-2939 Epub 2022/04/06

[9] Kirchdoerfer RN, Cottrell CA, Wang N, Pallesen J, Yassine HM, Turner HL, et al. Pre-fusion structure of a human coronavirus spike protein. Nature. 2016;**531**(7592):118-121 Epub 2016/03/05

[10] Millet JK, Whittaker GR. Host cell proteases: Critical determinants of coronavirus tropism and pathogenesis. Virus Research. 2015;**202**:120-134 Epub 2014/12/03

[11] Tortorici MA, Veesler D. Structural insights into coronavirus entry. Advances in Virus Research. 2019;**105**:93-116 Epub 2019/09/17

[12] de Groot RJ. Structure, function and evolution of the hemagglutinin-esterase proteins of corona- and toroviruses. Glycoconjugate Journal. 2006;**23**(1-2): 59-72 Epub 2006/04/01

[13] Neuman BW, Kiss G, Kunding AH, Bhella D, Baksh MF, Connelly S, et al.

A structural analysis of M protein in coronavirus assembly and morphology. Journal of Structural Biology. 2011;**174**(1):11-22 Epub 2010/12/07

[14] Binnicker MJ. Emergence of a novel coronavirus disease (COVID-19) and the importance of diagnostic testing: Why partnership between clinical laboratories, public health agencies, and industry is essential to control the outbreak. Clinical chemistry. 2020;**66**(5):664-666 Epub 2020/02/23

[15] Zhu N, Zhang D, Wang W, Li X, Yang B, Song J, et al. A novel coronavirus from patients with pneumonia in China, 2019. The New England Journal of Medicine. 2020;**382**(8):727-733 Epub 2020/01/25

[16] Holshue ML, DeBolt C, Lindquist S, Lofy KH, Wiesman J, Bruce H, et al. First case of 2019 novel coronavirus in the United States. The New England Journal of Medicine. 2020;**382**(10):929-936 Epub 2020/02/01

[17] Zhou P, Yang XL, Wang XG, Hu B, Zhang L, Zhang W, et al. A pneumonia outbreak associated with a new coronavirus of probable bat origin. Nature. 2020;**579**(7798):270-273 Epub 2020/02/06

[18] Chu DKW, Pan Y, Cheng SMS, Hui KPY, Krishnan P, Liu Y, et al. Molecular diagnosis of a novel coronavirus (2019-nCoV) causing an outbreak of pneumonia. Clinical Chemistry. 2020;**66**(4):549-555 Epub 2020/02/08

[19] Shen M, Zhou Y, Ye J, Abdullah Al-Maskri AA, Kang Y, Zeng S, et al. Recent advances and perspectives of nucleic acid detection for coronavirus. Journal of Pharmaceutical Analysis. 2020;**10**(2):97-101 Epub 2020/04/16

[20] Bustin SA, Nolan T. Pitfalls of quantitative real-time reverse-transcription polymerase chain reaction. Journal of Biomolecular Techniques: JBT. 2004;**15**(3):155-166 Epub 2004/08/28

[21] A. M. LAMP-Based Testing for COVID-19. Technology/Networks Industry Insight; 2020

[22] Poon LL, Leung CS, Tashiro M, Chan KH, Wong BW, Yuen KY, et al. Rapid detection of the severe acute respiratory syndrome (SARS) coronavirus by a loop-mediated isothermal amplification assay. Clinical Chemistry. 2004;**50**(6):1050-1052 Epub 2004/04/01

[23] Pyrc K, Milewska A, Potempa J. Development of loop-mediated isothermal amplification assay for detection of human coronavirus-NL63. Journal of Virological Methods. 2011;**175**(1):133-136 Epub 2011/05/07

[24] Mori Y, Nagamine K, Tomita N, Notomi T. Detection of loop-mediated isothermal amplification reaction by turbidity derived from magnesium pyrophosphate formation. Biochemical and Biophysical Research Communications. 2001;**289**(1):150-154 Epub 2001/11/16

[25] Shirato K, Yano T, Senba S, Akachi S, Kobayashi T, Nishinaka T, et al. Detection of Middle East respiratory syndrome coronavirus using reverse transcription loop-mediated isothermal amplification (RT-LAMP). Virology Journal. 2014;**11**:139 Epub 2014/08/12

[26] Hong TC, Mai QL, Cuong DV, Parida M, Minekawa H, Notomi T, et al. Development and evaluation of a novel loop-mediated isothermal amplification method for rapid detection of severe acute respiratory syndrome coronavirus. Journal of Clinical Microbiology. 2004;**42**(5):1956-1961 Epub 2004/05/08

[27] Njiru ZK. Loop-mediated isothermal amplification technology: Towards point of care diagnostics. PLoS Neglected Tropical Diseases. 2012;**6**(6):e1572 Epub 2012/06/30

[28] Shirato K, Semba S, El-Kafrawy SA, Hassan AM, Tolah AM, Takayama I, et al. Development of fluorescent reverse transcription loop-mediated isothermal amplification (RT-LAMP) using quenching probes for the detection of the Middle East respiratory syndrome coronavirus. Journal of Virological Methods. 2018;**258**:41-48 Epub 2018/05/16

[29] Craw P, Balachandran W. Isothermal nucleic acid amplification technologies for point-of-care diagnostics: A critical review. Lab on a Chip. 2012;**12**(14):2469-2486 Epub 2012/05/18

[30] Kawai Y, Kimura Y, Lezhava A, Kanamori H, Usui K, Hanami T, et al. One-step detection of the 2009 pandemic influenza A(H1N1) virus by the RT-SmartAmp assay and its clinical validation. PLoS One. 2012;**7**(1):e30236 Epub 2012/02/02

[31] Jeong YJ, Park K, Kim DE. Isothermal DNA amplification in vitro: The helicase-dependent amplification system. Cellular and Molecular Life Sciences: CMLS. 2009;**66**(20):3325-3336 Epub 2009/07/25

[32] Asai N, Nakamura A, Sakanashi D, Koita I, Ohashi W, Kawamoto Y, et al. Comparative study of SmartAmp assay and reverse transcription-polymerase chain reaction by saliva specimen for the diagnosing COVID-19. Journal of Infection and Chemotherapy: Official Journal of the Japan Society of Chemotherapy. 2022;**28**(1):120-123 Epub 2021/09/29

[33] Yamamoto K, Ohmagari N. Microbiological testing for coronavirus disease 2019. JMA Journal. 2021;**4**(2):67-75 Epub 2021/05/18

[34] Nagasawa S, Mori A, Hirata Y, Motomura A, Ishii N, Okaba K, et al. SmartAmp method can rapidly detect SARS-CoV-2 in dead bodies. Forensic Science International. 2022;**331**:111168 Epub 2022/01/10

[35] Serrano-Cumplido A, Ruiz Garcia A, Segura-Fragoso A, Olmo-Quintana V, Mico Perez RM, Barquilla-Garcia A, et al. Application of the PCR number of cycle threshold value (Ct) in COVID-19. SEMERGEN. 2021;**47**(5):337-341 Epub 2021/06/23. Aplicacion del valor umbral del numero de ciclos (Ct) de PCR en la COVID-19

Chapter 2

Real-Time qPCR and Rapid Antigen Testing of COVID-19 Testing: A Review and Comparison of Analytical Validity

Priya Hays

Abstract

Laboratory real-time qPCR (RT-qPCR) diagnosis and rapid antigen testing of COVID-19 variants have become a cornerstone of diagnosis of SARS-CoV-2 nucleic acids and antigens. This article proposes a comparative analysis of the benefits and limitations of these qualitative and quantitative methods through a literature review, and discusses how the validation of biomarker discovery in precision medicine could be applied to rapid antigen testing and molecular diagnostic workflows taking into considering testing sensitivity and specificity. Considerations of analytical validity and clinical validity arc a focus. Diagnostic accuracy as shown by ovcrall sensitivity and specificity of laboratory diagnostic RT-qPCR as compared with rapid antigen testing will be presented. This review is timely since the existing literature on RT-qPCR and rapid antigen testing for COVID-19 is significant containing large amounts of data, which at times is conflicting along with recommendations for streamlining these distinct methods for diagnostic testing of COVID-1 based on symptomatic presentation, vaccination and contact status. Since many cases currently are long COVID syndrome, the timeliness of the review may be paramount for potential future public health emergencies, especially involving respiratory illnesses.

Keywords: real-time qPCR, rapid antigen testing, sensitivity, specificity, biomarker discovery validation

1. Introduction

SAR-CoV-2 virus, the causative agent of COVID-19, led to a worldwide pandemic starting in 2020 and is still ongoing as result of novel variants. It is a positive-sense single stranded RNA enveloped virus that is responsible for causing a rapidly contagious respiratory illness through close human interaction. The pandemic as a result of the COVID-19 outbreak was declared on in March 2020 by the World Health Organization [1]. As of February 2023, worldwide incidence and mortality exceeded 600 million and 6 million respectively.

The viral genome and structure includes two ORF (1a and 1b) genes that code for RNA-dependent RNA polymerase, helicase and protease and four structural proteins including the nucleocapsid N, membrane N, envelope E and spike glycoprotein surface S. The RNA polymerase, ORF genes, E, N and S genes serve as targets for molecular testing through the RT-qPCR technique (**Figure 1**) [2, 3].

The functional receptor expressed on pulmonary epithelial cells, ACE-2 allows for the S protein to invade the host cell. The S protein is activated by cleavage, which leads to viral and host cell membrane fusion. The viral contents are emptied into the pulmonary alveolar epithelial cells and then the virus undergoes replication and the negative strand RNA is formed through RNA polyermase. The formed RNA strand serves as a template for the formation of positive RNAs which synthesize viral proteins in the cell cytoplasm, leading ultimately to viral particles that invade adjacent epithelial cells and potential infection via respiratory droplets through public transmission [4].

Efforts were directed to finding methods for diagnosis through tests that considered the virus' properties and its genome and structure. For acute infection, nucleic acid detection (RNA) became the gold standard for revealing infection. Literature

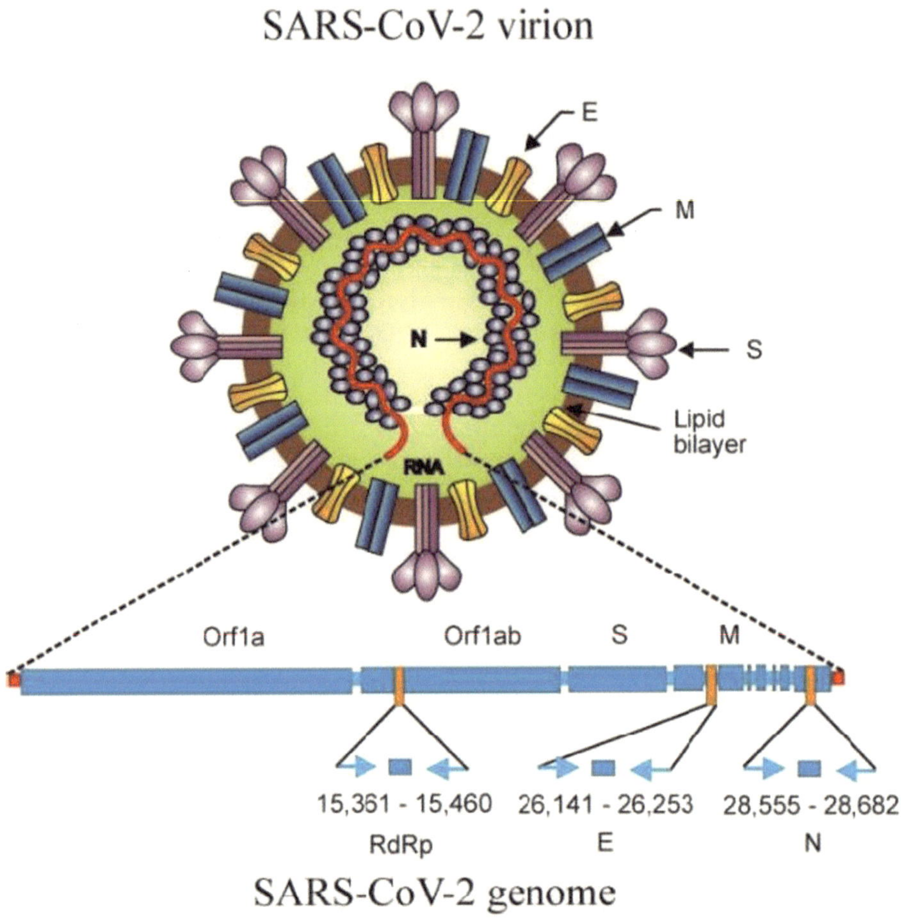

Figure 1.
Orf1a and Orf1ab and S and M genes (adapted from [2]).

on standard RT-PCR testing found that these tests were sensitive and specific but also time-consuming, which led to finding alternative approaches for timely, cost-effective in-house diagnostic kits based on antigen assays detecting viral antigen. A meta-analysis conducted in 2020 found variance in the accuracy of quantitative testing according to prevalence of COVID-19, with post-test probabilities decreasing according to prevalence (50%: 96%; 20%: 84%; 55%: 5%). Subsequent meta-analysis showed increased testing accuracy however the variation still persisted. According to Menesez, a number of factors in SARS-CoV-2 detection that involve preanalytical and analytical aspects of detection, such as delays, lack of standardization in specimen collection, assays that have not been adequately validated and poor storage conditions prior to arrival result in failure in testing accuracy. This is compounded by potential for procedure contamination, the disease period incubation and viral mutations [5]. According to Peeling et al., "a [rapid antigen] test should be specific enough to minimize the proportion of cases erroneously diagnosed as positive in low prevalence settings, and sensitive enough to avoid missing a diagnosis as COVID-19 prevalence increases" [6].

This chapter conducts a review of COVID-19 rapid antigen tests and real-time PCR amplification assays in terms of their sensitivity and specificity in the literature and compares the data, and provides the published recommendations in determining the appropriate testing according to clinical presentation and contact status in the form of algorithmic workflows. Currently, many commercial SARS-CoV-2 detection kits serve as the reference standards. This chapter also proposes the application of bio-marker discovery validation in precision medicine to COVID-19 laboratory molecular testing and rapid antigen testing.

2. Sensitivity and specificity for COVID-19 RT-PCR and antigen tests

The analytical validity of a diagnostic test is determined by the specificity and sensitivity of the assay. True positives are positives with the virus present; true negatives are negatives with the virus not present; false negatives are negatives with the virus present; false positives are positives without the virus present. Analytical validity and its referent to the rate of FP is seen the PPV of the test which mathematically is the PPV = TP/(TP + FP) x 100 and is the chance of disease upon receipt of a positive test and reflects disease prevalence, and specificity and sensitivity of the test [6].

2.1 Rapid antigen testing in asymptomatic and symptomatic COVID-19 patients: Emergency use authorization

A particle, fragment or molecule is considered an antigen whereby the immune system is triggered to produce antibodies to kill the pathogen. Rapid antigen testing in this context detects viral proteins, such as the S glycoprotein, M protein and the released N protein obviating the need for thermal amplification [1]. They reveal active viral infection and since antigens precede antibody and are targeted approaches, they do not reflect the recovery portion. Lateral flow assays or LFAs are considered the most commonly used rapid antigen testing for detection. The World Health Organization (WHO) recommended a minimum sensitivity of 80% and a minimum specificity of 97% for effective utilization of rapid antigen testing [7].

The analytical parameters of the Roche SARS-CoV-2 Rapid Antigen Test was determined by assaying negative and positive PCR samples and according to one study. 75 nasopharyngeal swabs from patients which tested SARS-CoV-2 RNA-negative were tested with the Real Star SARS-CoV-2 RT-PCR Kit "were collected and investigated using the SARS-CoV-2 Rapid Antigen Test, a lateral flow assay." The interpretation of lateral flow assays on samples showed that when both control line and test line were present, the test was regarded as SARS-CoV-2 antigen negative. When only the control line was present, the test was regarded as SARS-CoV-2 antigen negative. 75 positive nasopharyngeal swabs from patients that demonstrated huge variation in cycle thresholds and tested SARS-CoV-2 RNA positive with the Real Star SARS-COV-2 RT-PCR Kit were investigated using the SARS-CoV-2 Rapid Antigen Test cycle (Ct < 20: n = 5, Ct 20- < 25: n = 12, Ct25- < 30: n = 20, Ct 30- < 35: n = 29, Ct > = 35: n = 9). The specificity was determined as 96% and assay's "sensitivity with samples with a cycle threshold of < 25, 25 - <30, 30 - <35, and> = 35 was 100 %, 95 %, 44.8 % and 22.2 %, respectively." The authors note that these values are inferior to the PCR assay in terms of sensitivity and specificity but conclude that this alternative rapid antigen test is easier and more convenient to distinguish contagious from non-contagious individuals [8].

In 2021, a retrospective, cross-sectional study of an asymptomatic student population called StudyCov (n = 692) analyzed the specificity of the RT-PCR BioMerieux SAR-CoV 2 antigenic test. "The index test was the nasopharyngeal Abbott Panbio SARS-CoV-2 Ag rapid test" When stratified by symptoms and risk exposure, StudyCov revealed the following results:

- Overall sensitivity and specificity:
  - 65% [95%CI:49.0–76.4%]
  - 100% [95%CI:99.4–100%] respectively.
- In the asymptomatic sub-group:
  - 35% [95%CI: 15.4–59.2%] and 100% [95%CI: 99.3–100%] respectively.
  - "Using AT instead of RT-PCR, 13 (65%) subjects would have been missed, including 10 considered likely contagious."

The authors conclude: "This study shows the poor sensitivity of RAT (rapid antigen testing) in asymptomatic subjects, specificity being however excellent. The performance results fall below the World Health Organization recommendation of 80% sensitivity and question using AT in general population, especially when asymptomatic" [7].

Additional studies revealed the sensitivity and specificity of the Abbott BinaxNOW and Panbio test in asymptomatic patients. The evaluation of Abbott BinaxNow was conducted in asymptomatic walk-up patients and compared to RT-PCR: 3% had a positive RT-PCR. Sensitivity and specificity were respectively 93.3% (95% CI: 68.1–99.8%) and 99.9% (95% CI: 99.4–99.9%) for a Ct < 30 case definition. Unlike StudyCov, "the swab was done in both nostrils for both tests, the population was older and the AT was different," and "those differences might partly explain the performance differences". The Panbio SARS-CoV-2 AG Rapid Test Device with RT-PCR for emergency units-referred patients, 72.1% of which were asymptomatic. Sensitivity was 73.3% (95% IC: 62.2–83.8%) which is consistent with the BioMerieux results [9].

One field study conducted a rapid antigen detection test on infected individuals who were asymptomatic in an evaluation of the Panbio COVID Nasopharyngeal swabs were collected from household and non-household contacts. Confirmatory testing was done with the TaqPath Combo Kit using RT-PCR. They found that of 79 individuals tested positive by RT-PCR of whom 38 yielded positive RAD (rapid antigen detection) results. The overall sensitivity and specificity was 48.1% (95% CI 37.4–58.9) and 100%(95% CI 99.3–100), respectively, with sensitivity being higher in household (50.8%) than non-household contacts (35.7%); symptomatology presentation was more probable in RAT positive patients ($p < 0.001$). They conclude that "the Panbio test displays low sensitivity in asymptomatic close contacts of COVID-19 patients, particularly in non-household contacts. Nonetheless, establishing the optimal timing for upper respiratory tract collection in this group seems imperative to pinpoint test sensitivity" [9].

Table 1 shows the list as of September 2021 as compiled by Peeling et al. of rapid antigen tests and their sensitivities and specificities [6].

	Sample type	**Time of sample collection***	**Result reading**	**Sensitivity specificity†**	**Comments**
Abbott BinaxNOW, USA	Nasal swab	0–7 days	Visual, 15 min	97%, 99%	WHO Emergency Use Listing; US FDA Emergency Use Authorization; app for results; influenza A and B tests available
Abbott Panbio, USA	Nasal swab, nasopharyngeal swab	0–7 days	Visual, 15–20 min	93%, 99%	WHO Emergency Use Listing, US FDA Emergency Use Authorization pending
Access Bio CareStart, USA	Nasal swab, nasopharyngeal swab	0–5 days	Visual, 15-20 min	88%, 100%	US FDA Emergency Use Authorization
BD Veritor, USA	Nasal swab	0–5 days	Instrument, 30 min	84%, 100%	US FDA Emergency Use Authorization
LumiraDx, UK	Nasal swab	0–12 days	Instrument, 12 min	98%, 97%	US FDA Emergency Use Authorization
Quidel Sofia SARS Antigen Fluorescent Immunoassay, USA	Nasal swab nasopharyngeal swab	0–5 days	Instrument, 20 min	97%, 100%	US FDA Emergency Use Authorization; does not differentiate between SARS-CoV and SARS-CoV-2

	Sample type	Time of sample collection*	Result reading	Sensitivity specificity†	Comments
Quidel Sofia Flu and SARS Antigen Fluorescent Immunoassay, USA	Nasal swab, nasopharyngeal swab	0–5 days	Instrument, 20 min	95%, 100%	US FDA Emergency Use Authorization
SD Biosensor, South Korea	Nasal swab, nasopharyngeal swab	Not stated	visual, 15-30 min	97%, 100%	WHO Emergency Use Listing

Data from the Foundation for Innovative New Diagnostics.[2] *SARS-CoV = severe acute respiratory syndrome coronavirus. FDA = Food and Drug Administration. *Days after symptom onset.*
†Data from manufacturers.

Table 1.
Rapid antigen testing and sensitivity and specificity (adapted from Peeling [6]).

2.2 Sensitivity and specificity of quantitative real-time PCR COVID-19 diagnostic testing

When the pandemic cases were increasingly rising in early 2020, the nucleic acid amplification test quantitative real-time PCR began to serve as a major platform for the diagnosis of SARS-CoV-2 viral RNA [2].

Real-time PCR is a quantitative test that uses the principles of PCR for fast, accurate detection of the amplicon through the use of fluorescent dyes such as SYBRGreen and probes such as TaqMan. Viral RNA is reverse transcribed into cDNA which is then converted by Taq polymerase into double stranded DNA. Target genes detected by the amplification process included the ORF1ab EN, ORF1ab N and ORF1 ab NS "Viral load is determined through a threshold indicated by Ct level and quantified by levels of double stranded DNA indicated by fluorescence intensity" (**Figure 2**) [1].

When cases began to multiply at an increasingly alarming rate, real-time PCR emerged as the gold standard for diagnosis due to high sensitivity and specificity for symptomatic and asymptomatic carriers of infection. Banko et al. in [3] compared three real-time PCR tests and determined analytical sensitivity limit of detection at 500 copies/mL: The GeneFinder COVID-19 Plus RealAmp Kit (OSANG Healthcare Co., Anyang, Korea); Sansure Biotech (Sansure Biotech Inc., Changsha, China); TaqPath COVID-19 CE-IVD RT-PCR Kit (Thermo Fisher Scientific, Waltham, Massachusetts, USA), which amplify the ORF1ab and N genes. **Tables 2** and **3** show the positive and negative results out of 354 positive COVID-19 specimens. The authors conclude that there are similar analytical sensitivities and diagnostic accuracy. Final results indicated that the Sansure Biotech RT-qPCR method had significantly more positive results in comparison to the GeneFinder and TaqPath RT-qPCR methods ($p < 0.001$ and $p < 0.001$, respectively), and the GeneFinder RT-qPCR had significantly more positive results in comparison to the TaqPath RT-qPCR method (p 0.001 [3]).

Teymouri et al. stated that "Unlike other molecular tests that do not have perfect diagnostic specificity, qRT-PCR is highly specific with a specificity of almost 100 %" and "has led to RT-PCR becoming the gold standard molecular diagnostic test."

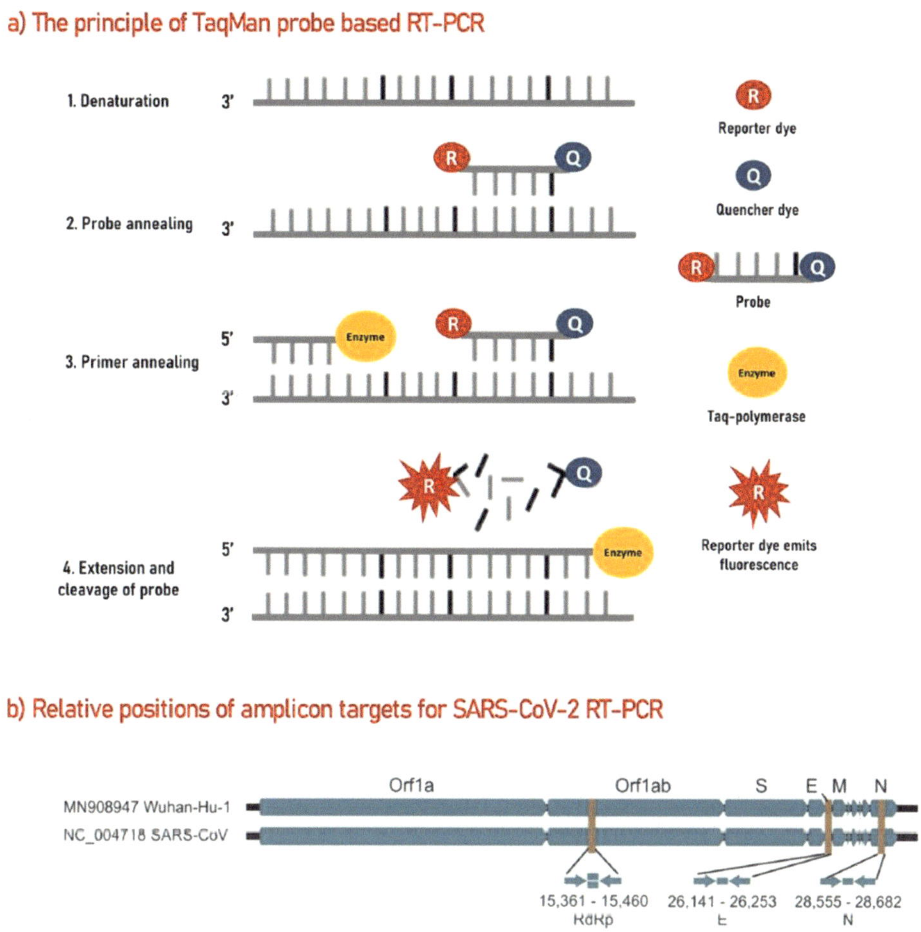

Figure 2.
Mechanism of quantitative RT-PCR method (adapted from [1]).

RT-qPCR Method	Target Gene	Positive, *n* (%)	Negative, *n* (%)
Sansure Biotech	Only ORFlab	4 (1.1)	350 (98.9)
	Only N	12 (3.4)	342 (96.6)
	Both ORFlab and N	190 (53.7)	164 (46.3)
Sansure Biotech final result		206 (58.2)	148 (41.8)
GeneFinder™	Only ORFlab	6 (1.7)	348 (98.3)
	Only N	11 (3.1)	343 (96.9)
	Only E	176 (49.7)	178 (50.3)
	Both ORFlab and N	176 (49.7)	178 (50.3)
GeneFinder™ final result		193 (54.5)	161 (45.5)

RT-qPCR Method	Target Gene	Positive, *n* (%)	Negative, *n* (%)
TaqPath™	Only ORFlab	0	354
	Only S	0	354
	Only N	24 (6.8)	330 (93.2)
	Both ORFlab and S	0	354
	Both ORFlab and N	132 (37.3)	222 (62.7)
	Both S and N	0	354 (100)
	ORFlab and S and X	22 (6.2)	332 (93.8)
TaqPath™ final result		178 (50.3)	176 (49.7)

Table 2.
RT-PCR tests comparison (adapted from [3]).

RT-qPCR Method	Measure of Diagnostic Accuracy with Its 95% CI						
	Sn (%)	Sp (%)	Overall Accuracy (%)	LR+	LR−	PPV (%)	NPV (%)
Sansure Biotech vs. Genefinder™	99.5 (98.5–1.00)	91.3 (87.0–95.7)	95.8 (93.7–97.9)	11.440 (6.94–18.87)	0.006 (0.001–0.040)	93.2	99.3
GeneFinder™ vs. TaqPath™	99.4 (98.3–1.00)	90.9 (86.7–95.2)	95.2 (93.0–97.4)	10.94 (6.86–17.45)	0.006 (0.001–0.044)	91.7	99.4
Sansure Biotech vs. TaqPath™	99.4 (98.3–1.00)	83.5 (78.0–89.0)	91.5 (88.6–94.4)	6.03 (4.33–8.42)	0.01 (0.001–0.05)	85.9	99.9

Table 3.
Diagnositc accuracy of RT-PCR tests (adapted from [3]).

However, pitfalls when the assay was being developed emerged in detecting true positives and true negatives in infected patients, and providers were counseled to combine molecular and clinical evidence. Sensitivity was reported at 45–60% in nasal swab samples and a false negative rate of 27% within the seven days when the illness onset in hospitalized patients. Patients diagnosed with chest CT scans and acute respiratory symptoms when molecularly tested on respiratory samples had a 33% false negative rate, as reported by researchers. This high false negative rate is attributed to variation in time of sampling since the onset of symptomatology, with values ranging from to 67% (day 1) to 38%, (symptom manifestation) and gradually returning to 66% on day 21 after symptoms have been observed (**Table 4**) [11].

RT-PCR results interpretation for the COVID-19 RT-PCR Single Plex Test kit by LabCorp shown in **Table 5** demonstrates that the test becomes "invalid" when the genes test negative. When the viral N genes test positive, the result displays "SARS-CoV-2 positive". The result is interpreted as "intermediate" when one only one of the target viral genes tests positive, requiring another testing. When all viral N genes test negative, the test result becomes "SARS-CoV-2 negative" [1].

Name of the Kit	Target Genes	Type	Sample Preparation	No. of Tests	Time	LOD	Sensitivity	Specificity	Cost (Per Test)
CovidNudge	rdrp1, rdrp2, E gene, N gene, n1, n2, and n3	RT-PCR	Automated	NA	~90 min	5 copies/μL	>94%	100%	GBP 10
Accula SARS-CoV-2 Test	N gene	RT-PCR	Automated	NA	~30 min	NA	100%	100%	USD 20
Cepheid Xpert Xpress SARS-CoV-2 assay	N2 and E	RT-PCR (real time)	Automated	10 per kit		0.02 PFU/mL			USD 19.8
FastPlex Triplex SARS-CoV-2 Detection Kit	ORFlab, N, RPP30	RT-dPCR	Manual	96 test per kit	90 min	285.7 copies/mL	>95%	95.7%	USD 1152
Gnomegen COVID-19 RT-Digital PCR Detection Kit	N1, N2	RT-dPCR	Manual	48 samples per day	180 min	2.5 copies per reaction	>95%	99%	NA
Bio-Rad SARS-CoV-2 ddPCR Test	N1, N2	RT-dPCR	Manual	96 samples	NA	400 copies/mL			NA
ePlexSARS-CoV-2 Test	N gene	End-point RT-PCR with electrochemical Detection	Automated	12 tests/kit	NA	1×10^3 copies/mL	99.02%	98.41%	NA

Table 4.
RT-PCR tests and sensitivity and specificity (adapted from [10]).

SARS-CoV-2 N1 (FAM)	SARS-CoV-2 N2 (FAM)	SARS-CoV-2 N3 (FAM)	RNAse P (FAM)	Interpretation	Report	Actions (Clinical Site Samples)	Actions (Pixel Home Collection Kit samples)
+	+	+	+/−	SARS-CoV-2 detected	DETECTED	Report results to sender and appropriate public health authorities	Report results to PWN Health, who will call the patient. Report the result to the appropriate public health authorities
If only one target is positive		+/−	+/−	SARS-CoV-2 Indeterminate	INDETERMINATE	The sample is repeated once. If results remain the same, it is reported to the sender as indeterminate and recommend recollection if the patient is still clinically indicated	The sample is repeated once. If results remain the same, it is reported to the sender as indeterminate to PWN Health, who will call the patient. Report the result to the Pixel Portal
—	—	—	+	SARS-CoV-2 Not Detected	NOT DETECTED	Report results to sender	Report result to PWN Health and the Pixel Portal
—	—	—	—	Invalid Result	INVALID	The sample is repeated once. If a second failure occurs, it is reported to the sender as invalid and recommend recollection if the patient is still clinically indicated	The sample is repeated once. If a second failure occurs, it is reported to PWN Health. Pixel's customer service will contact the patient to discuss options. Report the result to the Pixel Portal

Table 5.
Determination of validity of SARS-CoV-2 test (adapted from [1]).

2.3 Comparison and assessment of rapid antigen testing and real-time PCR

1000 types of molecular and antigen-based immunoassay tests are commercially available. According to one report, NAATs (nucleic acid amplification tests) such as RT-PCR can result in a positive test for weeks to months post infection, and may detect remnant viral RNA well after recovery. In contrast, antigen-based assays remain positive for 5–12 days subsequent to the onset of symptoms, and perform better in persons exhibiting a high viral load, which correlates with disease severity and death. Thus, rapid antigen testing may be a good indicator of potential transmissibility and correlate better than molecular tests with replication competent SARS-CoV-2 [12].

The rapid antigen tests are similar to PCR based tests in that detection is revealed during active viral infection rather than during the recovery situation. However, they are considered more reliable than antibody tests since they are target-specific. According to Yuce et al., "Antigen tests can be operated on LFA strip for rapid detection purposes or in ELISA format for better sensitivity, and high throughput uses (the simultaneous measurement of 96 samples)." A fluorescent immunochromatographic LFA assay for detecting the nucleocapsid (N) protein of SARS-CoV-2 was developed which "utilizes anti-N mouse antibodies and goat anti-rabbit IgG antibodies to create the test and control lines, respectively. It uses anti-N rabbit IgG marked with carboxylate-modified polystyrene Europium (III) chelate microparticles as signal particles" [1].

Repetitive RT-PCR testing has been shown to enhance performance characteristics, with false positive rates governed by differing factors, including time after onset of symptoms, symptom severity and nasal or oropharyngeal specimen used. **Figure 3** shows the timeline of viremia, antigenic and immunogenic response, illustrating the timepoints when the rapid antigen testing and RT-PCR are most sensitive. **Figure 4** illustrates a workflow whereby antigen and molecular testing can prove to be most

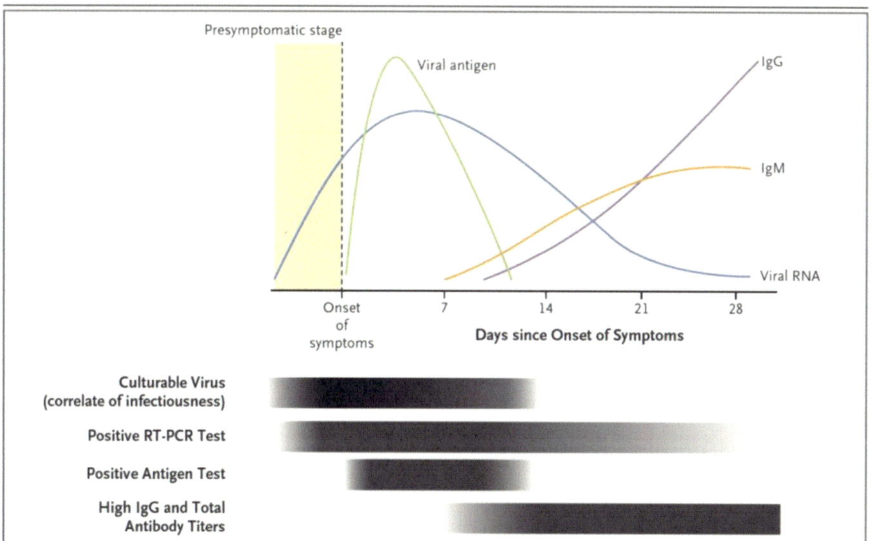

Figure 3.
Pathophysiology of viremia with positive molecular and rapid antigen tests output (adapted from [12]).

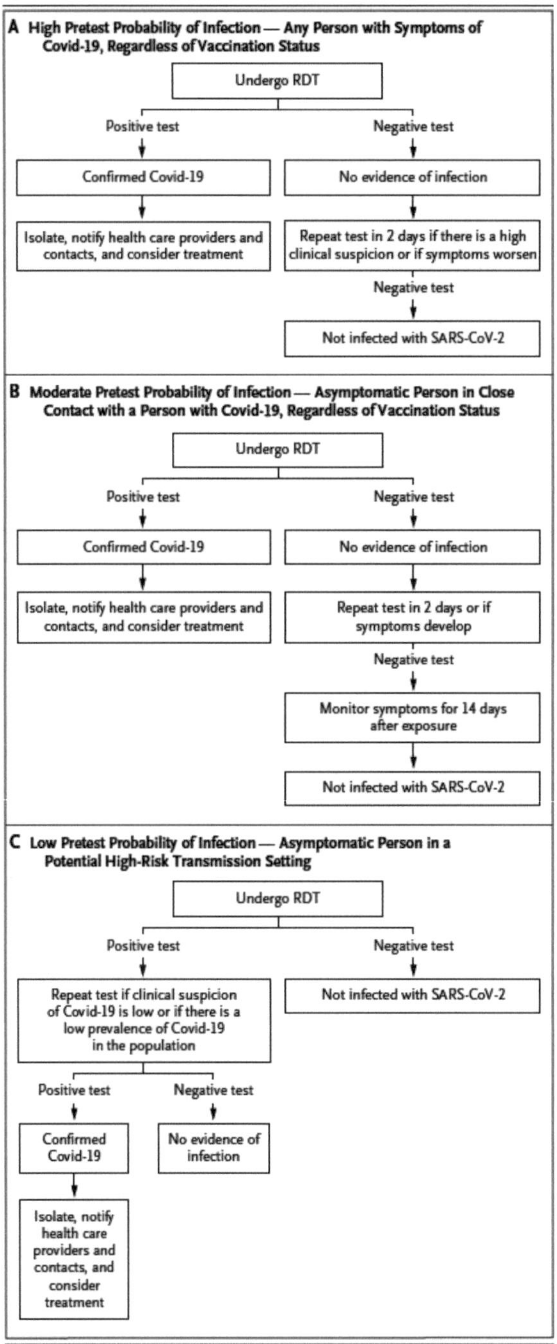

Figure 4.
Diagnostic testing workflows based on symptomatic status and patient management from diagnostic results (adapted from [12]).

accurate in the identification of the virus and resolution of symptoms, with different pathways for symptomatic and asymptomatic patients. When comparing the diagnostic tests, the predictive value of RT-PCR is higher and has higher post-test probability of reflecting the infected status of the individual, according to recent studies.

Pre-Analytical Assessment	• Clinical Presentation of COVID-19 symptoms • Determination of Quantitative Real-Time PCR Testing or Rapid Lateral Flow Antigen Testing • Well-defined population characteristics (disease incidence and prevalence) • Accuracy in sample collection and Collection in laboratory or home testing
Analytical Validation	• Laboratory personnel and calibration and maintenance of real-time PCR instruments • Enablement of rapid antigen kit for at-home convenient use • Assay predictive value: Quantitative comparison of Rapid Antigen Kit with "gold standard" RT-PCR Testing

Table 6.
Applying biomarker development validation guidelines to rapid antigen and molecular diagnostic testing (adapted from [13]).

3. Discussion: biomarker discovery validation and COVID-19 diagnostic testing

Analytical validation of biomarkers for use in genomic testing were developed and optimized for the sequencing of somatic samples, which became central to the implementation of precision medicine [13]. This paradigm can be adapted for COVID-19 molecular and rapid antigen testing for the purposes of streamlining sensitivity and specificity data. Pre-analytical and analytical validation criteria for biomarker validation may be applicable for COVID-19 testing. **Tables 6** is adapted from biomarker validation criteria and show how disease presentation and sample collection can lead to more accurate testing and better predictive value. The parameters in the second column show how assessment of pre-analytical characteristics, such as symptomatology, determination of test strategy, disease incidence and prevalence and accuracy in sample collection can form the basis of high analytical validity as determined by test choice of rapid antigen testing and compared with gold standard in asymptomatic and symptomatic individuals. Testing data generated can form the basis of high accuracy and evidence for analytical and clinical validation.

4. Conclusion

While the WHO announced the sensitivity criteria for rapid antigen testing, molecular testing remains the reference standard, despite logistical difficulties in personnel and laboratory instrument maintenance. Several studies have been performed comparing the two methods resulting in patient workflows as shown in recent reports. False negatives and false positives complicate the interpretative power of these tests, since erroneous clinical decisions would ultimately impact public health outcomes. Biomarker analytical validation can serve as a foundation for further streamlining of sensitivity of these results and possibly lead to more propitious control of pandemics.

Conflicts of interest

None to Declare.

Author details

Priya Hays
LLC, San Mateo, CA, United States

*Address all correspondence to: priya.hays@outlook.com

References

[1] Yuce M, Filizekin E, Ozkaya KG. COVID-19 diagnosis—A review of current methods. Biosensors and Bioelectronics. 2020;**172**:112752

[2] Artika IM, Dewi YP, Nainggolan IM, Siregar JE, Antonjaya U. Real-time polymerase chain reaction: Current techniques, applications, and role in COVID-19 diagnosis. Genes. 2022;**13**:2387

[3] Banko A, Petrovic G, Miljanovic D, Loncar A, Vukcevic M, Despot D, et al. Comparison and sensitivity evaluation of three different commercial real-time quantitative PCR kits for SARS-CoV-2 detection. Viruses. 2021;**13**:1321

[4] Parashar A. COVID-19: Current understanding of its pathophysiology, clinical presentation and treatment. Postgraduate Medical Journal. 2021;**97**:312-320

[5] Menezes S, Pestana DVS, Ferreira JC, Ribeiro de Carvalho CR, Felix MC, et al. Distinct outcomes in COVID-19 patients with positive or negative RT-PCR test. Viruses. 2022;**14**:175

[6] Peeling RW, Olliaro PL, Boeras DI, Fongwen N. Scaling up COVID-19 antigen tests: promises and challenges. The Lancet Infectious Diseases. 2022;**21**:e290-e295

[7] Ferte T, Ramel V, Cazanave C, Lafon M-E, Bebear C, et al. Accuracy of COVID-19 rapid antigenic tests compared to RT-PCR in a student population: The StudyCov study. Journal of Clinical Virology. 2021;**141**:104878

[8] Krüttgen A, Cornelissen CG, Dreher M, Hornef MW, Imohl M, Kleines M, et al. Comparison of the SARS-CoV-2 rapid antigen test to the real star Sars-CoV-2 RT PCR kit. Journal of Virological Methods. 2021;**288**:114024

[9] Torres I, Poujois S, Albert E, Colomina J, Navarro D. Evaluation of a rapid antigen test (Panbio™ COVID-19 Ag rapid test device) for SARS-CoV-2 detection in asymptomatic close contacts of COVID-19 patients. Clinical Microbiology and Infection. 2021;**27**:636.e1-636.e4

[10] Gupta N, Augustine S, Narayan T, O'Riordan A, Das A, et al. Point-of-Care PCR assays for COVid-19 detection. Biosensors. 2021;**11**:141

[11] Teymouri M, Mollazadeh S, Mortazavi H, Ghale-noie ZN, Keyvani V, et al. Recent advances and challenges of RT-PCR tests for the diagnosis of COVID-19. Pathology- Research and Practice. 2021;**221**:153443

[12] Drain P. Rapid diagnostic testing for SARS-CoV-2. New Eng. Journal of Medicine. 2022:1-9

[13] Hays P. Advancing Healthcare through Personalized Medicine. 2nd ed. Cham, Switzerland: Springer Nature; 2021

Chapter 3

Using Large Scale Rapid Antigen Testing (RAT) to Inform Participatory Ad-Hoc Community Surveillance for Emerging Communicable Disease Epidemics

Nicole Ngai Yung Tsang, Hau Chi So and Dennis Kai Ming Ip

Abstract

Besides the diagnostic use for infectious diseases in a point-of-care clinical settings, the simplicity and ease of self-performed RAT can also be an alternative approach for informing disease surveillance at the community level, carrying the potential advantage of enhanced timeliness, acceptability, and flexibility. Commissioned by the Hong Kong Government during the catastrophic fifth wave of the COVID-19 pandemic, our team established and maintained an ad-hoc large-scale participatory daily antigen rapid testing surveillance (DARTS) system for real-time situational awareness of SARS-CoV-2 activity to inform policy consideration in a timely manner. This Chapter will describe the concept and design of the surveillance approach, examine the practical feasibility and challenges, related logistical consideration on implementation and maintenance, technical aspects of data analysis to cater for the unique surveillance need, and other potential additional contribution of the data on understanding the novel disease (estimating vaccine effectiveness, and symptomatology and viral shedding pattern).

Keywords: rapid antigen test, surveillance, communicable diseases, epidemic, public health, community

1. Introduction

Since its emergence in late 2019, COVID-19 has caused unprecedented impact in terms of both mortality and morbidity in many countries. As of 8 February 2023, an estimated cumulative incidence of over 754 millions and mortality of more than 6.8 million were recorded globally [1].

As a novel infection causing the unprecedented global disease burden through successive rapidly evolving ways of epidemics in different countries, the painful experience from COVID-19 highlighted the need and importance of robust, timely, and representative community surveillance of novel and rapidly emerging communicable

IntechOpen

disease epidemics to guide a precise situational assessment and inform appropriate downstream public health strategy in an evidence-based manner. Although rapid antigen test (RAT) has been around for decades for different infectious diseases such as influenza and malaria, their use was limited mainly as a screening/diagnostic tool in a clinical point-of-care setting. With its rapid global popularization as a self-testing tool in the COVID-19 pandemic, the simplicity of the procedure and the ease of its usage has opened new opportunity for its use in a scaled manner in the community as an alternative approach for informing disease surveillance, which also offering the potential advantage of enhanced timeliness, acceptability, and flexibility.

This Chapter will give an overview of the concept of disease surveillance, discuss the inherent problems and difficulties of surveillance for novel and emerging epidemic disease, explore the potential for using RAT as a tool for enhancing disease surveillance, and basing on the experience of an ad-hoc RAT-based community surveillance system developed over two waves of the COVID-19 pandemic in Hong Kong to examine the feasibility and consideration of using RAT for surveillance during an evolving epidemic.

2. Concept of disease surveillance

2.1 Aim of surveillance

Public health surveillance is "the ongoing, systematic collection, analysis, and interpretation of health-related data essential to planning, implementation, and evaluation of public health practice" [2]. With appropriate analysis and interpretation, suitably collected surveillance can provide valuable data to inform the monitoring and action for disease control and prevention. Specifically, continuous surveillance over time allows for the monitoring of the temporal pattern of targeted infectious diseases among a population, so as to flag any abnormal change in disease activity in a timely manner (situational awareness) [3]. If allowable by the data granularity, stratified surveillance by geographic area or population subgroups would also allow for the pin-down of any aberration spatially or demographically. Moreover, when coupled with suitable additional data and analyses, well-collected surveillance data may also help to shed light on other important aspects of an emerging/novel infection, including risk factors and epidemiologic profile, disease burden, clinical disease symptomatology, and severity pattern, the effectiveness of vaccination or other public health interventions, and transmissibility and growth rate of the evolving epidemic.

2.2 Common approaches of infectious diseases surveillance

Surveillance can be conducted in two different ways, passive and active surveillance. Passive surveillance systems rely on the existing routine data reported from health facilities to the health agency. In active surveillance systems, public health workers take an active role to identify cases and monitor the population of interest, such as active calling and home visiting to follow-up individuals, thus significantly greater human and financial resources are required to depict a more comprehensive picture of disease burden and trends [3].

Different approaches have been commonly adopted for infectious diseases surveillance in a wide range of settings. In notifiable disease surveillance, practitioners are mandated to report cases of some pre-specified notifiable diseases of epidemic potential to the health agency, usually predefined by the World Health Organization, national or regional authorities. Routine administrative data, e.g. clinic/emergency room attendance and hospital admission episodes from public hospitals are another common statistics for passive surveillance. Syndromic surveillance can be conducted by examining syndromic groups of symptoms captured in an appropriate setting such as the emergency room, or using hospital billing data with ICD codes. Laboratory surveillance performed at reference laboratory can confirm the agent of infection, and monitor the disease incidence, and evolving trends of subtypes and variants of an infectious virus, and its infectiousness, seroprevalence [4].

Sentinel surveillance can also be conducted in designated sentinel sites in specific settings, such as general out-patient clinics, private clinics, associated health services centers to monitor the trends in general population; or in setting with high risk of outbreak such as child care centers, kindergartens, schools; or residential care home or elderly. Although conceptually distinct, active and passive surveillance for some important infectious diseases (e.g. seasonal influenza infection) are usually being performed in parallel in different community and health care settings to complement each other.

2.3 Important attributes of a surveillance system

Surveillance systems using different data in different settings are having important differences in a number of key characteristics, which ultimately affect their suitability in reflecting the changing disease activity and fulfilling surveillance needs for different stages and situations. Major important characteristics included representativeness, timeliness, sensitivity, and specificity.

Representativeness refers to the ability to give an accurate reflection of the epidemiological trend and disease burden in a defined population. For instance, data from sentinel out-patient clinics cover health care seeking activity in the general community while hospital admission data geared more toward capturing severe infections that need to be hospitalized. On the other hand, institutional data such as schools and care homes reflect more on the disease activity in those high risk setting, and may precede an increase in activity in the general community.

Timeliness refers to the ability of the system to issue signals efficiently to flag potential upsurge in community disease activity. Although it would be ideal for any changing disease activity to be alerted in a near real-time manner to inform situational assessment and the implementation of control measures, this relates to how effective and efficient the data collection/ analysis/and dissemination can be taken place, and carried non-trivial technical and logistical implications [4].

Specificity denotes clinically the reliable exclusion of people not having the infection or disease, while in a surveillance sense it refers to the ability to not flagging many false alarm of a change in disease activity when there is not any. This is an essential attribute to prevent overloading downstream manpower needed for follow-up and investigation of false negative signals, which may lead ultimately to desensitization and poor acceptance of the system.

There is generally a natural trade-off between data timeliness and data specificity. For instance, early data in the course of an infection (e.g. use of over-the-counter antipyretics/school absenteeism) tended to be very timely but being non-specific, while data in the later stage of a disease (e.g. clinical attendance/hospital admission/laboratory diagnosis) tended to be more specific but being much less timely. Earlier indicators also tended to better reflect disease activity in the community, including those mild infections without the need to attend medical care; while later indicators are generally geared more toward capturing patients in the more severe end of the clinical spectrum.

Sensitivity clinically represents the ability to accurately identify people having the disease, while in a surveillance sense it refers to the ability to flag a real change in disease activity when there is any. As all signals would need to be follow-up, choosing a suitable cut-off for flagging a signal would be an important consideration to strike a balance between the sensitivity and specificity when building any surveillance system.

2.4 Other issues to consider in building an effective surveillance system

Depending on the aims and objectives of surveillance, different systems would have their own sets of prioritized characteristics of high importance. Common issues crucial to build an effective surveillance system are discussed below [5].

2.4.1 Objective

A clear and specific objective is crucial for aligning the aim of surveillance and the planned uses of surveillance data with the parametrization of the systems. The disease, infection, or health event under surveillance should be specified with a predefined case definition. A consistent case definition throughout the surveillance period helps to monitor the temporal trend of the health event over time and avoid artifactually introduced change in observed disease activity.

2.4.2 Data source

A stable and reliable data source shall be identified to collect surveillance data in a timely and efficient manner. The legal, ethical, and privacy implication of data collation, collection, and management shall be considered, with proper informed consent if deemed necessary in an active system capturing personal data. For data to be reported from hospitals, clinics, or practitioners, or historic health records archived, a suitable streamlined and user-friendly automatic reporting system integrated with existing health information systems would help to enhance the availability, timeliness, and validity of surveillance data.

2.4.3 Sampling

After clearly defining the population under surveillance, the approach of data collection (sentinel or sampling) shall be decided. Theoretically, the data should be captured from a sample representative of the targeted population. The two commonest sampling strategies included random sampling, which helps to enhance representativeness; and convenient sampling which helps to improve participation for a quick establishment of the system. Other sampling consideration may include defining the catchment area for different districts to ensure a proper coverage of cases in different geographical locations. Depending on the purposes of the surveillance systems, the time period and intervals of the surveillance (continuous or intermittent, short term or long term) can be specified.

2.4.4 Frequency

The frequency of data collection is usually related to the targeted timeliness of the surveillance system to reflect the disease activity in the community. A short time interval with a frequent data collection, (e.g. daily or a near real-time system) may be necessitated for monitoring the trajectory of a rapidly evolving epidemic disease carrying huge public health implication. In practice, however, the optimal frequency of collecting data is also depended and limited by the sources and types of data, availability of the required reporting platform and manpower, and subject to different logistical and ethical constraints.

2.4.5 Data analysis

Data cleaning, collation, and management plan shall be prospectively planned and before the roll-out of surveillance. A proper process of data management, transfer, and storage should be chosen to ensure the validity of data and the compliance with applicable data security and confidentiality policy consideration. Important issue to decide on regarding the analysis methods included the frequency of analysis (hourly, daily, weekly, monthly), the detailed analysis algorithm, the need for standardization or stratified analysis, the cut-off threshold for issuing any alert signal and its performance in terms of sensitivity and specificity.

2.4.6 Dissemination

The results of the surveillance shall be disseminated to the relevant stakeholders and end users as feedback and to inform relevant downstream follow-up decisions and actions. A dissemination plan with detailed description of the frequency of result dissemination, mechanism of dissemination, targeted audience, and whether it matched and included all the recipients identified in the objectives set.

3. Unprecedented problems of surveillance for a novel emerging epidemic disease such as COVID

Comparing to regular surveillance systems used for routine ongoing situational assessment of infectious diseases such as seasonal influenza infection, the surveillance for novel/ emerging/evolving epidemic diseases such as COVID-19 pandemic, is much more complex and poses many unprecedented challenges and problems. A fundamental consideration would include how to make sure a robust surveillance data, either an existing routine one or some specific new data, can be maintained to inform a timely, specific, and stable surveillance [6]. Generally, the routinely reported daily case count of an infection may not be a good data stream for surveillance, especially during the midst of a rapidly changing epidemic.

3.1 The inadequacy of routine case count as a surveillance data

Although being routinely reported by most health authorities in different countries and smaller geographical sub-regions like provenances and cities, the daily PCR-confirmed case count, whether by self-collected deep throat saliva samples or professionally sampled specimens in a suitable clinical setting, carried major shortcomings for being used as a surveillance indicator. Being a lagging indicator [7], its timeliness can be affected by the turnaround time for laboratory confirmation, which can particularly be prolonged due to constrained testing capacity during periods of peak epidemic activity, when data timeliness is of utmost importance. Its general bias toward capturing infections in the more severe end of the clinical spectrum also affects the representativeness and ability to reflect prevailing disease activity in the general population [8].

3.2 Lack of consistency in case ascertainment

A consistent reporting pattern of disease episodes underlies the validity of any surveillance system, or else any change in observed disease activity may only reflect a varying testing/reporting/ascertainment practice [7]. As illustrated in the case of COVID-19, these can be a particularly serious problem during an emerging epidemic as case definition for infection and recovery can both vary widely between different health authorities and over time, such as whether probable or asymptomatic cases are officially counted [9, 10]. Inconsistency in reporting practice over jurisdictions has compromised the completeness and comparability of the surveillance data [11]. Spurious disease trend due to changing or update in case definition over time can also occur with evolving understanding about the new disease.

3.3 Issues of changing testing and reporting practice

Time-varying access to testing, medical consultations, and changing admissions to hospitals impeded the stability of a surveillance system using those data and thus its ability to monitor trends over time [7]. Changing testing criteria, policy, and arrangements can lead to a biased and inconsistent outcome capturing over the course of surveillance. Comparing to initial preference of laboratory-based PCR testing, the increasing availability and popularity of self-administered RATs testing can result in observed upsurge in observed disease incidence. Changing official testing policy over time, like the adoption or abandonment of mandatory/voluntary testing or the use of blanket testing as a community screening practice at different premises and subpopulations can also affect the observed temporal disease pattern. For a self-reported data such as symptoms or RAT testing result, changing reporting practice due either to concerns on downstream implication like isolation and quarantine, stigmatization, work or financial detriments can all affect the surveillance data.

4. RAT usage as point-of-care test

With its logistical simplicity of usage, more affordable cost, and wider availability, rapid antigen test (RATs) has become increasingly popular for identifying SARS-CoV-2 infection during the COVID-19 pandemic in a wide variety of clinical and community settings [12–14]. Common sampling methods included nasal swab and pooled throat and nasal swabs, either collected by healthcare workers or the general public. In contract to laboratory PCR testing requiring sample collection, storage, and transfer to laboratory, which typically associated with a turnaround time of one to several days, RAT has the advantage of giving a real-time result, and a much lower implication on expertise and laboratory processing capacity.

Previous studies have reported RAT to have a high positive predictive value, which makes it useful in setting of RAT as a self-testing tool, is particularly crucial to facilitate testing in remote areas with limited access to laboratory testing [15].

4.1 Usual setting and usage for clinical purposes

Over the course of the COVID-19 pandemic, RAT was being used for three main purposes. For symptomatic individuals presenting to a healthcare setting, RAT was being used as a point-of-case diagnostic tool to inform triage decision and clinical management [16]. For patients under isolation and exposed person in quarantine, RAT was also being used for self-monitoring to inform the discharge decision [17]. For other people in the community, RAT was widely used as a screening tool to establish eligibility for entering different vicinities like schools, hospitals, restaurants, recreational premises, and other governmental or private facilities. When laboratory testing capability was being stretched beyond the capability to cater for the testing demand, many jurisdictions had also shifted altogether from PCR to RAT as the official case definition of an infection.

Being sensitive, cost-effective, and portable RATs have been regarded a better performance than PCR in identification of infectious individuals [17].

4.2 Potential advantage of RAT for informing disease surveillance

Although being mainly used thus far as a diagnostic and screening tool, RAT also carried some potential advantages, including timeliness, specificity, and coverage for its potential use as a surveillance tool for the continuous monitoring of the epidemic/ pandemic disease activity in a community.

4.2.1 Timeliness

Although PCR-based case count was announced daily in many countries, it can be a very lagging indicator of the actual disease activity in the community, especially in areas having a limited laboratory testing capability and reserve. For RAT, as the test results of most brands are available within 20 minutes, this can minimize the turnover time required for specimen transfer and laboratory testing, and make it a suitable data to inform very timely or near real-time disease surveillance.

4.2.2 Specificity

From a systematic review examining the performance of RAT, high overall pooled specificity of 100.0% (95% CI = 98.8 to 100.0%) was reported among RATs for different COVID-19 variants [18]. Comparing to many traditional data being used for surveillance, including absenteeism, influenza-like illness, and other syndromic grouping, RAT result is having a much higher specificity for reflecting the ture activity pattern of the disease under surveillance by the system.

4.2.3 Coverage

As RAT can be easily performed by the general public, easy to manufacture and distribute, with wide availability in community settings, RAT can be readily accessible and conducted by individuals in remote areas, which helps to increase the coverage of testing on patient over the whole severity spectrum, and thus enhancing the representative of the surveillance system.

Among traditional surveillance data, there is generally an inherent trade-off between these three characteristics. More timely data are generally much less specific, and more specific data, like laboratory confirmed cases of influenza, are much less timely and reflecting covering those having more severe disease.

5. An example of RAT-based disease surveillance system for COVID-19

5.1 Background and context

Since its emergence in late 2019, COVID-19 has caused unprecedented impact in terms of both mortality and morbidity worldwide. The daily number of PCR-confirmed cases (case counts) represented the most fundamental data routinely reported in most countries to report the clinical and public health burden of COVID-19 during the evolving COVID-19 pandemic. However, its ability to accurately reflect the changing epidemic temporal trajectory in the community can be affected by many of the inherent bias of this data. These included its inherent bias toward preferentially capturing diseases over the more severe end of the clinical symptomatology spectrum or having an identifiable risk exposure, so that they would come forward for the PCR testing. In the contrary, self-performed RAT, because of its simplicity and high accessibility, may help to give a much more representative picture of the disease activity in the community when being used with an appropriate testing strategy. On the other hand, the better timeliness, flexibility, and scalability of RAT also facilitated its use in large-scale surveillance programme for informing situational awareness in an epidemic setting.

In this section, the feasibility and logistical considerations of using self-performed RAT to inform ad-hoc or regular disease surveillance in the context of a novel and evolving epidemic will be discussed, basing on the experience of a large-scale participatory Daily Antigen Rapid Testing Surveillance (DARTS) System, implemented to monitor the situation of COVID-19 in real time during the fifth wave of the COVID pandemic in Hong Kong.

In February 2022, Hong Kong was struck by its worse pandemic wave of COVID-19 with the Omicron variant (the fifth wave), which had caused an unprecedented impact and disruption to the societal functioning, healthcare delivery, and local economy. In particular, the sudden and rapid upsurge of case load had overwhelmed both the sampling manpower and laboratory capacity for PCR testing. The subsequent piling-up of specimens and the much prolonged turnaround time for diagnosis confirmation had jeopardized the timely implementation of downstream clinical management and public health measures, and had potentially contributed to the seedling of further transmission and disease propagation in the community. Commissioned by the Hong Kong Government during the catastrophic period, our team established and maintained an ad-hoc large-scale participatory daily antigen rapid testing surveillance (DARTS) system for real-time situational awareness of SARS-CoV-2 activity to inform policy consideration in a timely manner [19]. Established as an emergency ad-hoc public health initiative, the RAT-based disease surveillance system was aimed to provide a continuous, stable, and unbiased data for real-time situational assessment over the course of the SARS-CoV-2 epidemic in the local community in Hong Kong. Since its launch on March 3, 2022, the system has helped to track through the rapidly changing trajectory of the COVID-19 pandemic over its fifth and sixth wave of community activities in Hong Kong.

5.2 Practical considerations & challenges for implementation

5.2.1 Platform design

A suitable design of the surveillance platform should be chosen with a view to provide a robust results for reflecting the epidemic activity [20]. The collection of surveillance data for multiple time points generally adopts two common designs of observational study, serial cross-sectional and longitudinal cohort study [21].

Serial cross-sectional survey of samples drawn from the populations at multiple time points, though may be a practically and logistically simpler way to reflect the disease trajectory in the community, is subject to common problems of representativeness and comparability issues across samples involving different participants and with changing ascertainment practice over time [22, 23].

On the other hand, although cohort-based surveillance systems were logistically more challenging to build-up and maintain, the resultant representative cohort and the stable reporting behavior would be valuable in reflecting the temporal trajectory of an epidemic. The platform may also offer an opportunity for more detailed data to be collected for exploring various epidemiologic characteristics of the disease.

5.2.2 Recruitment

The lag-time required for the initial system setup of any ad-hoc surveillance system during the midst of an evolving and worsening epidemic is a crucial limiting factor on its ultimate utility. A simple and efficient recruitment approach should be adopted as far as possible to facilitate a speedy recruitment. A sufficient sample size would help to improve the precision and granularity of the data to allow for stratified monitoring of populations subgroups as defined by important demographic factors and geographical regions. On the other hand, although many surveillance systems are basing on convenience sample for the relative ease of recruitment, effort should always be paid to make sure the adopted recruitment approach, framework, and setting can help to enhance the representativeness of the sample to the general population, both in the beginning and over the course of the surveillance, or else a very biased intelligence may be resulted.

In our platform, a cohort of >10,000 individuals were recruited primarily by random digit dialing, which allowed the recruitment to be completed quickly and the system to be swiftly set up within a week. Representativeness of the cohort for the local population was ensured by adopting a pre-defined age-stratified quota, which was also statistically weighted in the calculation of the daily point prevalence. Dropouts and non-complying individuals were replenished by continuing recruitment to maintain the sample number and prevent surveillance fatigue.

5.2.3 The reporting procedure and details of information to be collected

As any concern regarding the workload and data privacy commitment would inevitably deter enthusiasm for participation, potential trade-off between the required data detail and hesitancy for participation should also be carefully considered. A realistic balance should be strived between any unnecessary obsession collecting a large amount of personal data against the potential impact on participation and compliance. In our system, besides the collection of basic demographic information and COVID-19 vaccination status in baseline, only a simple reporting of symptoms and the testing result was required on a weekly basis, which helped to minimize the excessive workload for result submission and privacy implication on participants.

5.2.4 Selection of test kit and quality consideration

RAT products of different assay brands may have very different technical complexity and variable sensitivity. To ensure a reasonable testing performance, the adopted RAT test kits should be meeting the World Health Organization's (WHO) priority target product profiles for COVID-19 diagnostics (i.e. sensitivity ≥80% and specificity ≥97%) and the United States Food and Drug Administration (FDA) Emergency Use Authorization (EUA). In our system, RAT kits of a single brand meeting the standard and with stable supply were chosen and provided to all participants to ensure the testing performance by minimizing potential misclassification as a result of suboptimal sensitivity and specificity.

5.2.5 Supply and distribution of test kits

During the midst of an evolving pandemic, accessibility of RATs can be a real problem. In our system, RATs for SAR-CoV-2 antigen were supplied to all participants on their consent to take part in the regular surveillance programme. Telephone hotlines were operated to address any enquiry and request for assistance.

Depending on the particular settings and scenario, a number of specific issues may need to be taken into consideration if testing kits were to be centrally supplied to participating individuals willing to take part in the surveillance to facilitate a rapid kick-starting of the programme. These issues may include the availability and stability of supply from the vendor, repacking needs subjecting to whether the supplied kits were originally in individual or bulk packing, and the logistical issues of test kit delivery to a large number of participants; each of those can become a non-trivial challenge given the community lockdown and/or infrastructure breakdown during the midst of an evolving epidemic.

5.2.6 Scheduling of testing to achieve regular data

A stable reporting behavior is the cornerstone of any useful surveillance data, as spurious temporal pattern can easily be resulted on changing reporting intensity as a result of surveillance fatigue or overzealous reporting. In our system, participants were being divided into seven cohorts of approximately equal size, with individuals in each cohort scheduled to perform the RAT on a designated day of the week irrespective of symptom or exposure history, so as to achieve a rolling testing schedule of around 1400 individuals on a daily basis.

5.2.7 Sampling and testing technique

In our system, RAT was performed by each participant, or sampled by parents for minors, with a self-sampled combined throat and nasal swab. Although the test is designed primarily for self-usage, our experience indicated that some people may still find it difficult to use and interpret, and the textual guidance provided in the pamphlet is difficult to understand and follow. In addition, there is also a potential problem of wrongly interpreting the testing results, especially among populations with advanced age and lower educational level. Simple instruction for the sampling and proper conduction of the self-tests, either for oneself or for minors, was therefore provided by us in both infographic format and step-by-step instructional video-clips specially recorded in-house by our team. Telephone hotlines were also operated to address enquiry and request for assistance from participants. Most individuals (99.22%) reported that they managed to successfully conduct the RAT testing independently under the video guidance.

5.2.8 Reporting platform

An in-house designed online platform was established to streamline direct enrolment and efficient registration of interested participants to the real-time surveillance system in a user-friendly manner. This online platform was also used for participants to report their demographic data initially and for the reporting of testing results and photos throughout the surveillance period through simple reporting steps. An individualized, password-protected account was assigned to each participating household for submitting their individual health records in a secured manner. To prevent any false positive due to reporting error, self-reported RAT positive results were validated with the RAT photos submitted on a daily basis.

5.2.9 Follow-up and cohort maintenance

Depending on the length of the targeted surveillance, proper maintenance of the surveillance cohort may be important to prevent surveillance fatigue when participants were losing interest or impetus on the regular testing and reporting activity, especially when their self-perceived risk was lowered with any apparent improvement in community epidemic activity. In our experience, following-up of participants regularly through phone calls, SMS, and WhatsApp was opined by the majority of our participants (98.96%) as useful for reminding them to complete the testing and reporting in a regular and timely manner. On the other hand, the operation of a responsive study hotlines would also be useful for addressing any problems that may be encountered by participants during the surveillance period.

5.2.10 Prospective data analysis

For many surveillance systems, including most seasonal influenza sentinel surveillance systems, analyzing on a weekly basis is generally good enough. Weekly or monthly data analysis with aggregated data across time would help to reduce data randomness and cyclical variability like weekend effects to give a more stable estimate over time. However, when more frequent data analysis (e.g. daily) is needed to inform a timely risk assessment and intelligence, the issue of data randomness may become a non-trivial. Data smoothing approaches, including random walk, simple moving averages, [24] exponential smoothing algorithm, or other algorithms [25], would help to remove noise due to random changes or seasonality, thus would help to avoid false alert and facilitate the identification real temporal trends of changing disease activity. The longer duration of data to be aggregated in the moving average, the more smoothed the data becomes, but may reduce the sensitivity and timeliness of noticing an increase in disease activity.

Depending on the types of surveillance data collected and the surveillance purposes, either the incidence or prevalence may be used. Incidence refers to the occurrence of new cases of disease or a health event in a population over a specified period of time, while prevalence refers to the proportion of a population who have an infection or a health event, including newly occurring cases and existing cases, in each specific time point or period. A repeated community-wide sampling without elucidating the information to differentiate new or existing infection would give an estimate of prevalence. Our system reported a simple daily point prevalence, estimated by dividing the number of individuals reported positive results by the number of individuals submitted valid test results on the same day. When allowed by available and collected demographic data, stratified analysis by gender, age group, geographical region, and socioeconomic status would help to assess the changing disease activity across different population subgroups and helps to assess potential differential risk and health care burden over an evolving epidemic. Longitudinal pattern of the changing infection prevalence over time would then allow the situational assessment of the changing epidemic situation, or calculating the effective reproductive number (Rt) to assess how quickly the virus is spreading in the community.

5.2.11 Feedback of surveillance intelligence

Timely and efficient feeding back of the surveillance intelligence in the most accessible manner is of utmost importance for informing any relevant community stakeholders and the general public regarding the evolving trajectory of the pandemic to facilitate appropriate downstream public health planning, decision-making, and action. In our system, the daily point prevalence of COVID-19 infection was disseminated on a real-time basis through an open online digital dashboard (https://covid19.sph.hku.hk/dashboard) to the general public and any potentially relevant stakeholders.

5.2.12 System evaluation

Evaluation of the system after it was up and running after a suitable period or stage would be important to assess how effective and efficient the system is, and to inform areas needing improvement. The Donabedian framework originally developed by the University of Michigan, involving an assessment of three categories: the "structure," "process," and "outcomes", represents a generic and useful framework for evaluating quality of health services and health care programmes [26]. In relation to a surveillance system, structure describes the context in which the system is built, process denotes the implementation and delivery of the surveillance steps, and outcomes refer to the effects of the surveillance intelligence on the understanding and handling of the evolving pandemic.

More specific, a more detailed evaluation of the nine key attributes of a surveillance system as listed below can be done using the CDC guidelines, which should be taken into consideration during both the planning and evaluation of any public health surveillance systems [27].

- **Simplicity** refers to the system's structure and ease of operation.
- **Flexibility** is the ability of the system to adapt to changing information needs and operating conditions with minimal additional cost.
- **Data quality** is the completeness and validity of the data collected through the system.

- **Acceptability** is the willingness of persons and organizations to participate in the system, including those who operate the system, report cases of the disease, or use the data.
- **Sensitivity** is the proportion of cases of a disease detected by a surveillance system and the ability of the system to monitor changes in the number of cases over time, such as outbreaks.
- **Predictive value positive** is the proportion of cases reported through the system that are accurately diagnosed instances of the disease under surveillance.
- **Representativeness** is the extent to which the system accurately describes the occurrence of the disease over time and its distribution in the population by place and person.
- **Timeliness** reflects the delay between steps in a surveillance system and availability of information for control of the disease under surveillance when needed.
- **Stability** is the ability of a surveillance system to collect, manage, and provide data without failure and to be operational when needed.

Evaluation of the surveillance system after landmark stages is important and can inform the way forward in relation to the evolving epidemic. Our evaluation based on the Donabedian framework and CDC guideline had revealed the surveillance initiative to be a representative, stable, and timely surveillance system with high data quality and acceptability.

5.3 Conclusions

The successful establishment and maintenance of the DARTS system during the SARS-CoV-2 pandemic in Hong Kong demonstrated that results of regular self-performed RAT in the community can be used to inform situational awareness of the trajectory of an evolving epidemic as an ad-hoc participatory surveillance system. Our experience also demonstrated that it is logistically and technically feasible for establishing such a large-scale ad-hoc surveillance platform in a timely manner during an emergency, including the recruitment, follow-up, and maintenance of a sizably large number of representative surveillance participants with good compliance. The regular non-symptom and risk-based testing approach helped to give a more representative picture of disease activity of all severity spectrum, including subclinical cases who still carried an implication of downstream transmission. The use of RAT instead of PCR has helped to avoid the constraint of manpower and testing capacity, which the government has also quickly adopted for case definition.

Acknowledgements

This project was supported by the Henry Fok Foundation and a special commissioned fund (reference number COVID-19FHB, COVID-19HHB) from the Health Bureau of the Hong Kong Special Administrative Region Government. We acknowledge research support by Jerome Leung, Grace Ng, Oscar Kwok, Christine Ning, Kenny Mok, Clarice Guo, and Kaki Chen.

Conflict of interest

The authors declare no conflict of interest.

Author details

Nicole Ngai Yung Tsang, Hau Chi So and Dennis Kai Ming Ip*
WHO Collaborating Centre for Infectious Disease Epidemiology and Control, School of Public Health, Li Ka Shing Faculty of Medicine, The University of Hong Kong, Hong Kong SAR, China

*Address all correspondence to: dkmip@hku.hk

References

[1] WHO. Weekly Epidemiological Update on COVID-19 - 8 February 2023 2023 [updated 8 February 2023]. Available from: https://www.who.int/publications/m/item/weekly-epidemiological-update-on-covid-19---8-february-2023

[2] Gregg M, Gregg MB. Field epidemiology. USA: Oxford University Press; 2008

[3] Murray J, Cohen AL. Infectious disease surveillance. In: International Encyclopedia of Public Health, 2nd ed. Vol. 4. 2017. pp. 222-229

[4] Hopkins RS. Design and operation of state and local infectious disease surveillance systems. Journal of Public Health Management and Practice. 2005;**11**(3):184-190

[5] World Health Organization. Division of Emerging and other Communicable Diseases Surveillance and Control, Zimbabwe. Ministry of Health and Child Welfare & Liverpool School of Tropical Medicine. Protocol for the Evaluation of Epidemiological Surveillance Systems. World Health Organization; 1997. Availabe from: https://apps.who.int/iris/handle/10665/63639

[6] Rolka H. Analytical challenges for emerging public health surveillance. CDC's Vision for Public Health Surveillance in the 21st Century. 2012;**61**:35

[7] Fox SJ, Lachmann M, Tec M, Pasco R, Woody S, Du Z, et al. Real-time pandemic surveillance using hospital admissions and mobility data. Proceedings of the National Academy of Sciences. 2022;**119**(7):e2111870119

[8] Alwan NA. Surveillance is underestimating the burden of the COVID-19 pandemic. The Lancet. 2020;**396**(10252):e24

[9] WHO. Public Health Surveillance for COVID-19: Interim Guidance. 2022. Available from: https://www.who.int/publications/i/item/WHO-2019-nCoV-SurveillanceGuidance-2022.2

[10] US Centers for Disease Control and Prevention. Coronavirus Disease 2019 (COVID-19): about CDC COVID-19 data. 2020. Available from: https://www.cdc.gov/coronavirus/2019-ncov/cases-updates/about-us-cases-deaths.html

[11] Gold JAW, DeCuir J, Coyle JP, Duca LM, Adjemian J, Anderson KN, et al. COVID-19 case surveillance: Trends in person-level case data completeness, United States, April 5–September 30, 2020. Public Health Reports. 2021;**136**(4):466-474

[12] Centers for Disease Control and Prevention. Guidance for SARS-CoV-2 Rapid Testing Performed in Point-of-Care Settings. 2022. Available from: https://www.cdc.gov/coronavirus/2019-ncov/lab/point-of-care-testing.html

[13] WHO. Advice on the Use of Point-of-Care Immunodiagnostic Tests for COVID-19. 2020. Available from: https://www.who.int/news-room/commentaries/detail/advice-on-the-use-of-point-of-care-immunodiagnostic-tests-for-covid-19

[14] Australian Government. COVID-19 Point-of-Care Tests. 2022. Available from: https://www.tga.gov.au/products/covid-19/covid-19-tests/covid-19-point-care-tests

[15] Boum Y, Eyangoh S, Okomo M-C. Beyond COVID-19 — Will self-sampling and testing become the norm? The Lancet Infectious Diseases. 2021;**21**(9):1194-1195

[16] Bond KA, Smith B, Gardiner E, Liew KC, Williams E, Walsham N, et al. Utility of SARS-CoV-2 rapid antigen testing for patient triage in the emergency department: A clinical implementation study in Melbourne, Australia. The Lancet Regional Health - Western Pacific. 2022;**25**:100486

[17] Routsias JG, Mavrouli M, Tsoplou P, Dioikitopoulou K, Tsakris A. Diagnostic performance of rapid antigen tests (RATs) for SARS-CoV-2 and their efficacy in monitoring the infectiousness of COVID-19 patients. Scientific Reports. 2021;**11**(1):22863

[18] Kim J, Sung H, Lee H, Kim JS, Shin S, Jeong S, et al. Clinical performance of rapid and point-of-care antigen tests for SARS-CoV-2 variants of concern: A living systematic review and meta-analysis. Viruses. 2022;**14**:1479, 1-17. DOI: 10.3390/v14071479

[19] DKM I, NNY T, Leung CW, Ng KY, So HC, Cowling BJ, et al., editors. Daily antigen rapid testing surveillance (DARTS) system for COVID-19 - a large-scale ad-hoc participatory community surveillance initiative using self-performed lateral flow rapid antigen tests in Hong Kong. In: OPTIONS XI for the Control of Influenza; 2022 September 26-29. Belfast, UK: The International Society for Influenza and other Respiratory Virus Diseases (isirv); 2022

[20] Butler AE, Battista K, Leatherdale ST, Meyer SB, Elliott SJ, Majowicz SE. A comparison of repeat cross-sectional and longitudinal results from the COMPASS study: Design considerations for analysing surveillance data over time. International Journal of Social Research Methodology. 2022;**25**(5):597-609

[21] Cerón A, Ortiz MR, Álvarez D, Palmer GH, Cordón-Rosales C. Local disease concepts relevant to the design of a community-based surveillance program for influenza in rural Guatemala. International Journal for Equity in Health. 2016;**15**(1):69

[22] Martijn PFB. A comparison of efficiencies of longitudinal, mixed longitudinal, and cross-sectional designs. Journal of Educational Statistics. 1986;**11**(3):171-181

[23] Setia MS. Methodology series module 3: Cross-sectional studies. Indian Journal of Dermatology. 2016;**61**(3):261-264

[24] Hyndman RJ. Moving Averages. In: Lovric M, editor. International Encyclopedia of Statistical Science. Berlin, Heidelberg: Springer Berlin Heidelberg; 2011. pp. 866-869

[25] Arabzadeh R, Grünbacher DM, Insam H, Kreuzinger N, Markt R, Rauch W. Data filtering methods for SARS-CoV-2 wastewater surveillance. Water Science and Technology. 2021;**84**(6):1324-1339

[26] Donabedian A. An Introduction to Quality Assurance in Health Care. Oxford, England: Oxford University Press; 2002

[27] German R, Lee L, Horan J, Milstein R, Pertowski C, Waller M. Guidelines working group Centers for Disease Control and Prevention (CDC). Updated guidelines for evaluating public health surveillance systems: Recommendations from the guidelines working group. MMWR - Recommendations and Reports. 2001;**50**(RR-13):1-35

Chapter 4

Rapid Test and Chagas Disease: An Overview

Marcelle Almeida Caminha,
Ana Luiza Barbosa Godart Cavalcante
and Rubem Figueiredo Sadok Menna-Barreto

Abstract

Chagas disease (CD) is an infectious illness with great socioeconomic impact. Historically, it has mainly affected the poor population in Latin America. However, globalization sets a new scenario, featuring an increasing CD incidence worldwide especially due to parasite transmission by infected blood in non-endemic countries. Noteworthily, CD is predominantly marked by a subclinical progression, so that for most cases, the correct diagnosis may take years, even decades, post-infection. Public actions such as active search of infected people and donors screening are imperative for both identification of individual health assistance and disease control. Nonetheless, the main affected areas lack laboratory infrastructure, resource, and specialized personnel, making the use of conventional immunoassays unfeasible. Moreover, parasite genetic variability and cross-reaction with close-related infectious diseases impose a stringent diagnosis algorithm. Thus, although rapid tests are a great option, its applicability is still restricted in the context of this disease. In this regard, this chapter will discuss the use of immunochromatographic-based assays for CD, their limitations, and perspectives. The performance of commercially available kits in comparison to the conventional serologic tests will be also debated, covering their antigen selection, origin of population studied, and type of samples.

Keywords: Chagas disease, *Trypanosoma cruzi*, screening, diagnosis, rapid test, immunochromatography

1. Introduction

Chagas disease (CD) is a systemic illness caused by the hemoprotozoan *Trypanosoma cruzi* [1]. Its classical infection route is vectorial, depending on the contact of the vertebrate host with triatomine bugs' feces containing the parasite [1]. Nowadays, oral infection plays an important role in CD transmission, especially in the Amazon region. Such a route also comprises a vector-dependent pathway, and it may take place upon ingestion of food or beverage contaminated by an infected insect [2, 3]. Therefore, CD has mainly affected the low-income population of rural areas where the favorable conditions for the triatomines are usually found intra or peridomiciliary, hence contributing to its establishment as endemic in Latin America [4]. Notwithstanding, while its incidence has been historically close related to socioeconomic and cultural factors, immigration has set a new epidemiological scenario [4–6]. Consequently, the profile of the infected people and at risk of acquiring the infection currently also includes population in urban centers, especially those from non-endemic countries, where the transmission occurs mostly by blood transfusion, solid organ transplantation, and from mother-to-child [5, 6].

Its clinical manifestations generally take years, or even decades, to occur and are predominantly related to chronic cardiac and/or gastrointestinal tissue damages, which are commonly associated with fibrosis and ganglion impairment [7]. Noteworthily, although only 30–40% of those infected present chronic signs and/or symptoms, its severity and incapacitation are enough to cause a global annual cost ranging billions of dollars (US$) owing to healthcare assistance and loss of productivity [8–10]. Thus, the propagation control of *Trypanosoma cruzi* infection is imperative.

In this regard, it is important to stress out that initiatives from Latin American countries, mainly based on vector control and screening of donors and pregnant women, resulted in a reduction of at least 62% of *T. cruzi* infection over the past 30 years [4, 10, 11]. However, the low rate of successful CD diagnosis (<10%) persists as a major obstacle to the interruption of infection dissemination [12]. Notably, two main factors are associated with disease diagnosis hindrance: (i) education of healthcare workers and technical training concerning CD aspects and detection of infection—especially in non-endemic regions, and (ii) the subclinical and slow-paced disease progression [13, 14]. To put it another way, the risk of infection remains permanent, or even greater in the case of non-endemic countries, because most people are oblivious to their own infection status, either due to a long-lasting asymptomatic clinical state, incorrect diagnosis, or lack of *T. cruzi* screening policies. Ergo, the majority of CD carriers do not receive the correct treatment.

The CD chemotherapy is based on only two drugs: benznidazole and nifurtimox. The efficacy of both nitroderivatives is greatly influenced by patient's age and disease phase, so the sooner the medicines are taken, the higher the chances of cure [15, 16]. This is extremely important, as both drugs present limited activity in the chronic phase, especially in the symptomatic stage, besides severe side effects that commonly result in treatment abandonment [15, 16]. Public health initiatives are crucial to improve and increase early diagnosis rate and, consequently, timely treatment. However, in the meantime, CD remains the predominant cause of infectious cardiomyopathy in Latin America and a great burden in non-endemic countries [6, 17].

2. Standard methods and protocols for CD diagnosis

CD is marked by an acute and chronic phase, each with specific aspects that reflect the diagnostic methods of choice. Given that the onset of infection is characterized by a high parasitemia, the techniques related to direct parasite detection on peripheral blood by light microscopy comprise the gold standard for diagnosis during the acute stage, including in cases of congenital infection [18, 19]. Thus, the methods mainly applied are thin, thick, or fresh blood films. Alternatively, concentration methods, such as Strout and microhematocrit, may be employed [18, 19]. These protocols are especially indicated for the diagnosis of congenital infection and can be performed with either umbilical cord or venous blood from neonates and infants [20]. Polymerase chain reaction (PCR) can also be used, however, it should preferably be carried out within the first and third months of life [20]. In addition, serological follow-up is indicated for infected infants as well as for those with negative direct parasite detection with an infected mother. This analysis should be performed from the eighth month of life, when maternal IgG is no longer detected [20, 21].

In contrast, the chronic phase features a subpatent parasite load. In this sense, indirect detection methods that rely on parasite amplification, such as hemoculture, xenodiagnosis, and PCR, may be performed [19]. However, these tests show low sensitivity at this stage, so that a negative result has poor conclusive value to discard infection [19]. As the end of the acute phase is accompanied by seroconversion, the chronic stage is characterized by a continuous production of IgG. Ergo, diagnosis of suspected cases of long-lasting infections is predominantly based on immunoassays. Nevertheless, there is no gold standard or reference test since none of the kits commercially available exhibit ideal performance regarding both sensitivity and specificity [19]. Consequently, at least two tests must be performed, so that infection is either confirmed or ruled out only if both assays present the same profile of reactivity (positive or negative, respectively) [18]. Hence, when inconclusive results are obtained, another test must be carried out [18]. The immunoassays applied must necessarily differ in terms of either detection principles or antigenic set and present complementary sensitivity and specificity [18]. Furthermore, in the absence of a biomarker for cure, conversion to non-reactive profile in subsequent tests in an interval of time has been considered a parameter to confirm the parasite elimination by trypanocidal treatment [22].

Although indirect hemagglutination (IHA) and indirect immunofluorescence (IIF) are frequently used, enzyme-linked immunosorbent assay (ELISA) is the most employed method, once (i) it is better suited for large-scale analysis and (ii) presents a considerable variety in terms of antigenic preparations [23]. In addition, chemiluminescent microparticle immunoassay (CMIA) and western are also recommended, the latter mainly employed as a confirmatory assay and/or discriminatory test in inconclusive cases [18, 19].

ELISA kits are produced with either (i) whole parasite extract, (ii) semi-purified fractions, (iii) recombinant proteins (full-length or chimeras), or (iv) synthetic peptides—the latter two being commonly used as multiplexed formulations. Alternatively, combining purified homogenate with recombinant proteins is employed as well [23]. This flexibility is a major advantage given that test reactivity may vary according to sample origin due to host genetic background and/or differences among parasite strains. As a matter of fact, *T. cruzi* presents a wide genetic variability, so that populations are classified into six groups named discrete typing units (DTU) TcI-VI and Tcbat [24], which exhibit different geographical prevalence [25, 26]. Moreover, the diversity of ELISA kits also covers the necessary arrangement of sensitivity and specificity complementation. In this regard, the implementation of recombinant proteins and synthetic peptide have shown to improve test accuracy by reducing cross-reactivity with other diseases, especially leishmaniasis [19].

Noteworthily, the protocol for the screening process in blood banks and prenatal care—as a health policy measure to reduce *T. cruzi* infection dissemination—rely on the application of a single immunoassay, which must present a high sensitivity. In this context, ELISA and CMIA are the main recommended methods [18]. Nonetheless, in case of a positive result, another test must be carried out to confirm the diagnosis.

3. Applicability of rapids tests and its perspectives in CD context

Considering that those most affected by CD are from either remote areas or small towns with low resource in developing countries, the main immunoassays used for diagnosis and screening purposes do not meet the reality of local points of care, which commonly lack the needed infrastructure and the specialized personnel [27]. Furthermore, field studies are also hampered, as these tests are usually performed with plasma or serum obtained from venous blood extraction [28]. Thus, even if the assay is not carried out locally, transport of materials and equipment for sample adequate handling and storage are still required, as well as a trained team, which often translates in logistic complexity and, ultimately, in higher cost. More importantly, depending on the notification system applied, patient acknowledgment regarding their results is not safely guaranteed when the tests are performed latter on. Consequently, there is a patent demand for rapid tests [29], which have as basic concept a cheap and fast assay, with an easy development that ideally eliminates the necessity of specialized technicians, equipment, including in terms of sample manipulation, and cold storage, enabling their use on-site [30].

The World Health Organization and the Pan American Health Organization's guidelines consider rapid tests as an alternative screening method for ELISA only in the context of seroepidemiological studies [18]. Their use is not recommended for clinical diagnosis or screening in hemotherapy services based on (i) the detection variation, (ii) the increased false negative rate (2–7 per 1000) in comparison to the association of two conventional serological methods for diagnosis of chronic patients and (iii) the cost-effectiveness, especially when there is a high demand, such as in blood banks [18].

Nonetheless, in 2005, the Chagas National Program of Bolivia incorporated the use of a specific rapid test (Chagas Stat-Pak, Chembio Inc.) as the frontline method in both clinical practice and seroepidemiological surveys [31]. Notably, Chagas Stat-Pak (CSP) has shown sensitivity and specificity ranging from 93.4 to 100.0% and from 97.3 to 99.3%, respectively, among Bolivian municipalities [28, 31–33]. However, to follow the recommended diagnosis algorithm, positive cases still must be confirmed by a conventional immunoassay [31]. In this sense, studies have shown promising results regarding the synchronous combination of two rapid tests with different antigen composition as an alternative strategy for definitive diagnosis in low-resources settings in Bolivia, Argentina, and Colombia [28, 31, 34–37]. The association of two rapid tests displayed ≥93.3% of diagnostic efficiency when using results obtained by at least two conventional immunoassays as reference [28, 31, 35, 36]. This alternative protocol has a great advantage in speeding up the process of patient continued medical assistance, especially regarding the offer of trypanocidal drugs and, eventually, other necessary treatments. In line with that, the combination of rapid testing with electrocardiogram (ECG) performed by a mobile device was also evaluated in Bolivia [38]. Interestingly, out of the 25 people with ECG abnormalities compatible with chagasic chronic cardiomyopathy, 22 (88%) presented a positive profile on the rapid test. As per the current protocol, the diagnosis of these patients was later confirmed by ELISA. ECG was carried out in a device connected to a smartphone and processed by a medically certified app; the exams were performed by non-physicians in a remote area, however, within 24 h the data were analyzed, and results were reported by cardiologists located overseas [38]. Taking into account the lack of clinical tools for patient's progression monitoring toward symptomatic stage [22, 39–41], the incorporation of already known potential protein markers for such questions, especially those for early cardiac impairment [42, 43], in rapid test is an appealing and strategical approach to improve the assistance of individuals infected and should be addressed in the near future.

In view of congenital transmission, rapid testing has also been evaluated in Latin American pregnant women, mainly at the time of delivery [44–48]. This practice has a great impact on disease control when the mother was not tested during prenatal care, once trypanocidal efficacy is high and well tolerated by infants [20, 48]. Surprisingly, reported data indicates that a rapid test outperformed ELISA assays [45, 46]. Furthermore, aiming to investigate the recovery time of newborns infected congenitally and submitted to trypanocidal treatment 1 day after birth, Chippaux et al. [21] monitored periodically the level of specific anti-*T. cruzi* antibodies by ELISA; newborns without infection, but with an infected mother were included as control. From the eighth month, the authors carried out rapid testing in parallel to the conventional assay. At the ninth month, none of the patients showed immunoreactivity in the rapid test, while 12% remained testing positive by ELISA. Within the following 7 months, all of these patients presented antibodies titres below the ELISA cut-off [21]. This delayed seronegativity may be related to the extended set of antigens and/or the different epitopes components of the ELISA kit in comparison to the rapid test used. Moreover, anti-*T. cruzi* IgG originally from the mother was not detected in the mentioned control group since the fifth month despite the continued breastfeeding [21]. Conversely to the observed in infants, Jackson et al. [49] still detected reactivity in 2 ELISA assays and in the same rapid test when applying sera from adults of endemic regions after 3 years of treatment with nifurtimox.

Up on the released data reporting rapid tests performance on endemic population, a health center in Geneva, Switzerland, sought to study its feasibility regarding the screening of Latin American immigrants [50]. The majority of infected individuals was from Bolivia, and as a result of the rapid testing agreement with the conventional immunoassays and reproducibility, it was incorporated at the hospital as a point-of-care test in both the primary care center and the maternity ward (testing at delivery) [50]. In Italy, a different test has shown high specificity and was used as a third assay for evaluation of samples with discordant results [51], while in Spain, a rapid test was applied to screen co-infection in Latin Americans immigrants diagnosed with HIV [52].

4. Performance of immunochromatographic rapid tests commercially available

As previously mentioned, parasite and/or host genetic background may be related to reactivity discrepancy. Thereby, it is strongly suggested that the rapid test is field validated in the area of interest before officially incorporating its use [31, 35]. This process should ideally be carried out at a national level by encompassing different sites [31], once circulating strains may vary from one region to another within the endemic countries [24, 25]. Thus, this topic is focused on the main marketed rapid tests with reported performance studies (**Table 1**).

These assays are based on the detection of anti-*T. cruzi* antibodies circulating in the bloodstream upon recognition of recombinant proteins (**Figure 1**). In the absence of a gold standard immunoassay, conventional serology methods have been used as reference to evaluate rapid test performance (**Table 2**). Generally, the tests can be carried out with small volumes (5 to 100 μL) of either plasma, serum, or whole blood (**Table 1**). However, the latter comprises the best working sample type as it does not require further processing and, in the case of immediate testing, it may be obtained from fingertip puncture, perfect for the context of the field research. Moreover, the results are obtained within 10–35 min (**Table 1**).

CSP detection capability relies on the recognition of the recombinant antigens B13, 1F8, and H49/JL7 [53]. Notably, it has been trending as the most evaluated rapid test in

Rapid test	Antigen	Sample	Vol. (μL)	RT (min)	SS (%)	SP (%)	Sample origin	Ref.
Chagas Stat-Pak (Chembio)	B13, 1F8 and H49/ JL7	S or P WB	5 10	15	93.4 to 100.0	97.3 to 99.3	Bolivia	[28, 31–33]
					100.0	100.0	Colombia	[35]
					97.1 to 100.0	94.8 to 99.9	LATAM[1]	[53, 54]
					87.2 to 96.0	93.2 to 99.9	LATAM[2]	[34, 50, 56]
Trypanosoma Detect (InBios)	ITC8.2	S or P WB	10 20	10	84.8	97.9	LATAM[1]	[62]
					89.6 to 92.9	94.0 to 100.0	LATAM[2]	[56, 64]
Chagas Detect Plus (InBios)	ITC8.2	S or P WB	10 20	20	96.2 to 100.0	87.1 to 99.3	Bolivia	[28, 31, 60]
					100.0	99.1	Colombia	[35]
Simple Stick Chagas (Operon)	Pep2, TcD, TcE and SAPA	S	35	10	92.4 to 100.0	91.6 to 92.4	LATAM[2]	[67, 68]
Simple Chagas WB (Operon)	Pep2, TcD, TcE and SAPA	S or P WB	10 NS	10	84.9 to 92.5	70.7 to 96.8	LATAM[2]	[56, 67, 70]
SD Bioline Chagas Ab (Standard Diognostics)	1F8 and H49	S, P or WB	100	15	97.6 to 100.0	93.8 to 97.7	Argentina	[36, 37]
					90.7	94	LATAM[2]	[56]
WL Check Chagas (Wiener Lab)	NS	S, P or WB	40	25–35	87.3 to 93.4	98.8 to 100	Argentina	[36, 37, 74]
					88.7	97	LATAM[2]	[56]
OnSite Chagas Ab Combo (CTK Biotech)	NS	S or P WB	20 40–50	15	90.1 to 95.5	91.0 to 96.9	LATAM[2]	[56, 68]
Chagas Instantest (Silanes)	NS	S or P	10	15–25	76.6	79.0	LATAM[2]	[56]
TR Chaga* (Bio-Manguinhos)	IBMP-8.1 IBMP-8.4	S	5	15	100.0	100.0	Brazil	[75]

Sensitivity (SS) and specificity (SP) ranges are displayed based on the overall results obtained in the studies mentioned. Vol: volume; RT: reaction time; S, P, and WB: serum, plasma, and whole blood, respectively; LATAM: Latin America; NS: not specified.
[1]*Studies performed at endemic regions that included samples from at least two different countries.*
[2]*Studies that incorporated surveys of Latin American samples in non-endemic regions.*
**Type of sample, volume, and reaction time were informed as described in the respective reference.*

Table 1.
Rapid test commercially available for CD diagnosis that present performance reports in the literature.

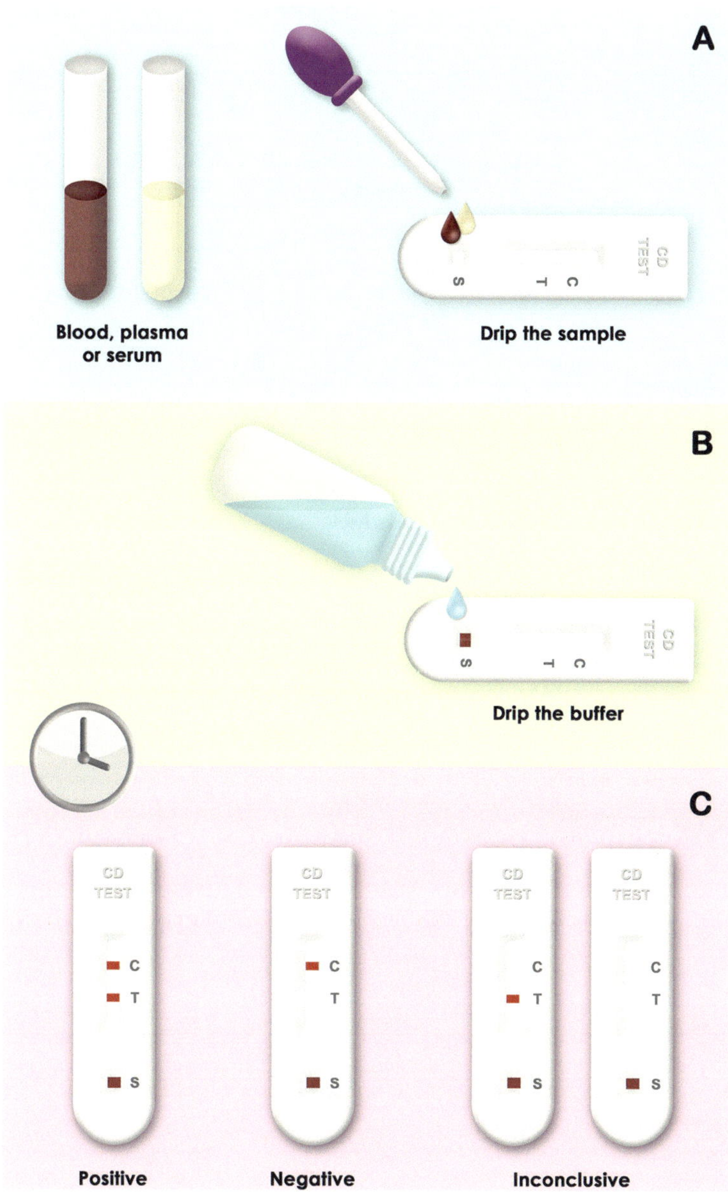

Figure 1.
Rapid testing scheme. (A) Either plasma, serum or whole is placed onto the sample site (S) and after (B) the addition of buffer, the molecules flow laterally through the membrane by capillary. (C) Within minutes, the results are obtained and can be interpreted by naked eye. Those positive comprise at least two bands, referring to the control line and the antigen detected by the anti-Trypanosoma cruzi IgG. Notably, the test can have more than one epitope separated in different reaction areas. A result is stated as negative when only the control line is apparent, and an assay is determined as inconclusive when the control line is not detected.

both field and clinical seroprevalence studies, including in non-endemic countries. By using serum as testing sample, CSP has shown sensitivity ranging from 97.1 to 100.0%, and specificity from 94.8 to 99.9% among populations from South and Central Americas [53, 54]. Surprisingly, reactivity of samples from Midwest and Northeast

Conventional immunoassay	Principle	Antigen	Rapid test	Ref.
Bioelisa Chagas (Biokit)	ELISA	TcD, TcE, Pep 2 and TcLo1.2	CSP, SSC, OnSite, SCWB, SD Bioline	[50, 57, 68–70, 73]
Certest (BiosChile)	ELISA	Lysate (Tulahuén and Mn strains)	SSC, OnSite	[68]
Chagas III (BiosChile)	ELISA	Parasite lysate	CSP, CDP, TD, TR Chagas	[35, 62, 75]
Chagas IgG + IgM I (Vircell)	ELISA	FRA, B13 and MACH[a]	CSP, CDP, TD	[35, 64]
Chagas HAI-Immunoserum (TIIC)	IHA	NS	CSP	[53]
Chagas Polychaco (Lemos Lab.)	IHA	NS	CSP, CDP, TD, WL Check Chagas, SD Bioline	[31, 32, 36, 60, 63, 65, 74]
Chagatest v.2.0 (Wiener)	ELISA	Parasite lysate	CSP, TD, CDP	[28, 31–34, 60, 63]
Chagatest v.3.0 (Wiener)	ELISA	Pep 1, 2, 13, 30, 36, and SAPA	CSP, CDP, TD, SD Bioline	[28, 31–34, 44–46, 54, 60, 65, 66, 73]
Chagatest (Wiener)	IHA	Pep 1, 2, 13, 30, 36, and SAPA	SD Bioline	[73]
Chagatek (Lemos Lab.)	ELISA	Purified antigens	CSP, CDP	[28]
Elecsys Chagas (Roche Diagnostics)	E-CLIA	Recombinant proteins	TD	[64]
ELISA cruzi (bioMérieux)	ELISA	Parasite lysate	CSP, TD, SSC, OnSite	[50, 62, 68]
Gold ELISA Chagas (Rem Diag.)	ELISA	Recombinant proteins and purified lysate	TR Chagas	[75]
Hemagen Chagas (Hemagen Lab.)	ELISA	Purified antigens	CSP, CDP, TD	[34, 44, 66]
IFI Chagas (Bio-Manguinhos)	IFI	Strain not specified	TR Chagas	[75]
ID-PaGIA2 (DiaMed)	GA	Ag2 and TcE	SSC, OnSite	[68]
ID-PaGIA3 (DiaMed)	GA	Ag2, TcE and TcD	SSC, OnSite	[68]
Ortho *Trypanosoma cruzi* (Ortho-Clinical Diag.)	ELISA	Parasite lysate	CDP, SSC, OnSite, SCWB	[66, 68, 69]
T. cruzi IgG (BLK Diag.)	ELISA	Parasite lysate	SSC, OnSite	[68]
—	IIF	Parasite Tulahuén strain	WL Check Chagas, SD Bioline	[36]
In-house[b]	ELISA	Parasite lysate (Y strain)	CSP	[53]
	ELISA	Parasite lysate (Peru strain)	CSP	[54]
	ELISA	Parasite lysate (H1 strain)	CSP	[46]

Conventional immunoassay	Principle	Antigen	Rapid test	Ref.
	ELISA	Parasite lysate (Tulahuén strain)	TD, WL Check Chagas, SD Bioline	[37, 62]
	ELISA	Parasite lysate (PM strain)	TD	[62]
	ELISA	Parasite lysate (Mc, T and Dm28 strains)	SSC, OnSite, SCWB	[67, 68]
	ELISA	Parasite lysate	SCWB	[69, 70]
	ELISA	Parasite lysate (MHOM/CO/06/338)	SD Bioline	[73]
	IIF	Parasite Y strain	CSP	[53]
	IIF	Parasite Colombian strain	CSP, CDP	[35]
	IIF	NS	CDP	[60]
	IIF	Parasite Tulahuén strain	TD, WL Check Chagas, SD Bioline	[62, 37, 74]
	IIF	Parasite Mc, T and Dm28 strain	SSC, OnSite, SCBW	[67, 68]
	IHA	NS (Tulahuén strain)	TD	[62]
	IHA	NS (PM strain)	TD	[62]
	IHA	NS	WL Check Chagas, SD Bioline	[37]
	TESA-blot	Secreted/excreted proteins (Y strain)	CSP, CDP	[34]
	Western blot	Parasite lysate (H1 strain)	CSP	[46]

Those applied as confirmatory are also included [45, 57, 65, 69]. ELISA: enzyme-linked immunosorbent assay; E-CLIA: electrochemiluminescence immunoassay; GA: gel agglutination; IHA: indirect hemagglutination; IIF: indirect immunofluorescence; CSP: Chagas Stat-Pak; CDP: Chagas Detect Plus; TD: Trypanosoma detect; SSC: simple stick Chagas; SCWB: simple Chagas WB; SD Bioline: SD Bioline Chagas Ab; OnSite: OnSite Chagas Ab Combo; NS: not specified; TIIC: Tecnologia Imunológica Indústria e Comércio.[a]Recombinant protein composed by Pep 2, TcD, TcE and SAPA antigens.
[b]Methods without clear reference of a commercial kit were considered as in-house assays.

Table 2.
Conventional immunoassay used as reference to evaluate rapid test performance.

regions of Brazil resulted in 98.5 and 94.8% of sensibility and specificity, respectively [53], even though the epitope B13 is derived from a 140 kDa protein detected in the surface of Y strain trypomastigotes [55], which belongs to one of the predominant DTUs in the respective area [24, 25]. Furthermore, sera from El-Salvador displayed the lowest sensitivity (97.1%) [53]. In a multicenter study carried out by Sánchez-Camargo et al. [56] with sera tested in national reference laboratories for Chagas disease diagnosis located in Brazil, Argentina, Colombia, Costa Rica, Mexico, United States of America, France, Spain, and Japan, the CSP exhibited 87.2 and 93.2% of sensibility and specificity, respectively [56]. On average, 50 samples (ca. of 25 positive and 25 negative) per region were analyzed, however, neither the origin of the donors sorted by each facility in non-endemic areas nor the correspondent data per country was discriminated. The reduced performance was accounted to sera selection, which comprised samples stored for averagely 2 years and with moderate to low reactivity profiling. The later aspect is of major importance, once one cannot rule out that methods used for sample reactivity classification could vary among the laboratories enrolled [56]. Curiously, this study also reported a lower sensitivity when using plasma in comparison to serum, while two other studies have demonstrated high level of agreement (99.7–100.0%) among different sample types (sera stored with or without 50% glycerol, plasma, whole blood and/or eluates from filter paper containing dried whole blood) [50, 53]. In this regard, CSP exhibited outstanding results (100.0% for both sensitivity and specificity) in whole blood testing in Colombia [35].

Interestingly, analysis of CSP in surveys of Latin Americans living in non-endemic countries showed a predominant seroprevalence in Bolivian immigrants [34, 50, 57]; sera testing presented low performance [34], while whole blood accused a sensibility and specificity of 95.2 and 99.9%, respectively, being 97.2% of the positive results from Bolivian origin [50]. By the time the CSP was implemented as a diagnostic tool by the Bolivian Ministry of Health, only one of the studies conducted so far had included samples from such region (n = 21) [53]. Therefore, since then, studies have been done to evaluate and field validate CSP performance in different Bolivian sites. Most of these works used whole blood for the CSP testing and either serum or plasma for conventional serological assays taken as reference. As previously mentioned, detection performance varied among municipalities, with sensibility and specificity ranging from 93.4 to 100.0% and from 97.3 to 99.3%, respectively [28, 31–33]. Noteworthily, lower sensitivities were obtained by Roddy et al. and Chippaux et al. when working with age groups ranging from 9 months to 17.9 years old (93.4%) and from 11 to 20 years old (89.2%), respectively [32, 33]. More worrisome, up to 7.6% of discrepancy between CSP and ELISA results was observed in women pregnant either at the moment or in the preceding 3 years at the time of the respective study [33]. Nevertheless, the same Chagatest v.3.0 (Wiener) failed to detect infection in 29.5% of women PCR-positive at delivery, while the overall CSP rate of false negative was 9.6% [45]. This research enrolled women from Argentina, Honduras, and Mexico, which displayed 97.3, 96.1, and 67.3% of CSP reactivity, respectively [45]. Although the detection in Mexican women was expressively reduced, CSP still outperformed the ELISA assay applied by 39.4% [45]. In a lower-prevalence scenario in Mexico, by taking western blot as confirmatory test, Gamboa-Léon et al. [46] demonstrated similar results between CSP and Chagatest v.3.0 (Wiener), especially in samples collected from umbilical cord.

Both the *Trypanosoma* Detect (TD) and Chagas Detect Plus (CDP) are based on the multiepitope recombinant protein ITC8.2 [58]. Produced by InBios, their main differences reside in product format and clearance by the U.S. Food and Drugs Administration agency. While TD is presented as a dipstick with application restricted to research [59], the CDP consists of an improved version [60], designed in cassette format—with the gold conjugate maintained in liquid solution—and is marketed for diagnostic use in the USA [60, 61].

TD evaluation in sera samples from Argentina, Ecuador, Mexico, and Venezuela resulted in 82.5, 84.3, 77.5, and 95.0% sensitivity, respectively. On the other hand, specificity was high, with the lower result detected in Ecuador (95.6%) and the greater in both Mexico and Venezuela (100.0%) [62]. In the work by Sánchez-Camargo et al. [56] previously mentioned, it presented an overall sensitivity and specificity of 92.9 and 94.0%, respectively. Similar sensitivity was observed in Bolivian women at delivery (92.7%), however, a higher specificity was shown (99.0%) [63]. In addition, regarding the same study performed with PCR-confirmed infected women with whole blood also collected at delivery in Argentina, Honduras and Mexico, TD testing resulted in more cases of seroreactivity in comparison to ELISA Wiener (v. 3.0) in samples from the latter two countries, while no difference was observed for those from Argentina [45]. Given that the ELISA kit used and the TD share 4 epitopes (peptides 1, 30, 36 and SAPA) between their sets of antigens [58], the TcF and Kmp-11 peptides included in the latter test may be related to the differential detection observed. Nonetheless, CSP still outperformed TD in both Honduras and Argentina [45]. In a survey of immigrants from endemic countries living in Spain that included an electrochemiluminescence immunoassay as reference, a lower sensitivity was obtained (89.6%) with whole blood, while excellent specificity was maintained (100.0%) [64]. Notably, such reference test (Elecsys Chagas, Roche Diagnostics) does not share any antigen with TD.

Aiming to increase sensitivity, the TD was modified, resulting in the CDP assay [60]. Its first performance evaluation was carried out with paired sets of whole blood and sera samples from Bolivian populations encompassing adults (with or without heart disease), pregnant women at delivery and children up to 17 years old. Tests results obtained with each type of sample displayed 90.3% of agreement, with whole blood showing a reduced sensitivity (96.2 vs. 99.3%) and higher specificity (98.8 vs. 96.9%) [60]. Following studies testing whole blood from individuals in different regions of Bolivia reported sensitivity of 92.1–100.0% and specificity of 87.1–99.3%, being the best results obtained in a high seroprevalence area [28, 31, 65]. In Colombia, CDP showed an outstanding performance with whole blood testing as CSP (≥ 99.1% for both parameters) [35]. Interestingly, reported data of Latin American CDP testing in the USA points to difference of performance between plasma and serum, with greater relevance for those from Mexico and Central America (mostly represented by El-Salvador) [34, 66]. More importantly, CDP showed superior sensitivity to samples from these same regions in comparison to three others conventional serological assays (two ELISAs and one IHA), whereas a lower specificity (87.5–92.3%) was observed in the overall analysis [66].

Simple Stick Chagas (SSC) and Simple Chagas WB (SCWB) also comprise rapid tests elaborated in two different formats that are based on the same antigen, a chimeric recombinant protein that englobes the peptide 2, TcD, TcE and SAPA epitopes [67] (**Table 1**). The former has a dipstick design and can be used with serum, while the latter is displayed as a cassette and can be carried out with either whole blood, plasma, or serum [67]. Studies that include these tests were mainly centered in evaluating their applicability as screening tool of Latin American immigrants and others with epidemiological background of risk living in Spain [67–70]. Sera testing with SSC showed 92.4–100.0% of sensitivity and 97.9% of specificity, which is reduced to 91.6–92.4% when considering cross-reactivity [67, 68]. As for whole blood testing with SCWB, peripheral samples exhibited a 92.1 and 93.6% of sensitivity and specificity, respectively [67]. Interestingly, capillary samples obtained by finger prick displayed a performance of 86.4 and 95% for the respective parameters [67, 71]. In these works, the onsite results were confirmed latter on by conventional immunoassays carried out with samples collected and stored on filter paper [67, 71]. On the other hand, a 92.5% of sensitivity was observed by Chejade et al. [70] when working with capillary blood and confirmatory assays done with samples frozen until use. Poorer performance was observed by Sánchez-Camargo et al. [56] when testing sera with SCWB, which displayed an overall of sensitivity and specificity of 84.9% and 70.7%, respectively, and a variable response in the quality control evaluation among the laboratories. Authors also called attention to misguiding instructions in the manufacture datasheet, which reflected in the outcome. However, such errors were already corrected [72]. Finally, little to no cross-reactivity was observed for leishmania with SSC and SCWB, however, both assays showed relevant number of false-positives with samples from individuals infected with malaria [67, 68].

The SD Bioline Chagas Ab rapid test relies on the recognition of recombinant antigens H49 and 1F8 (**Table 1**). Although Sánchez-Camargo et al. [56] reported 90.4 and 94.0% of sensitivity and specificity, respectively, in Colombia, this assay presented a great potential value for diagnosis confirmation when using sera (100.0% specificity), but not as a screening tool [73]. Nonetheless, in Argentinean adult population, sera and whole blood testing presented satisfactory sensitivity (97.6–100%), whereas better specificity was achieved with the latter type of sample (93.8 vs. 97.7%) [36, 37]. WL Check Chagas (WLC) was used in parallel in both studies, which reported similar results [36, 37]. Adding up to other works, WLC is more suitable as a confirmatory test regardless of the type of sample used, especially in Argentina (≥ 98.8% of specificity) [36, 37, 56, 74].

Performance data of Chagas Instantest, OnSite Chagas Ab Combo, and TR Chagas is scarce, beginning with the antigenic formulations (**Table 1**). Except for the last one, all rapid tests were analyzed by Sánchez-Camargo et al. [56], which—for the best of our knowledge—consists of the only independent source of information for Chagas Instantest. This assay showed sensitivity of 76.6% along with a specificity of 79.0% [56]. A moderate agreement was detected between the obtained and expected results, besides a bad profile and reproducibility on the quality control evaluation [56]. Moreover, authors reported a high frequency of invalid tests and a strong background color, making a clearer interpretation difficult [56]. As for the OnSite Chagas Ab Combo, sera testing presented 90.1–95.5% of sensitivity and 91.0–96.9% of specificity and displayed cross-reactivity with samples from individuals with either leishmaniasis or malaria [56, 68]. At last, a prototype version of TR Chagas was evaluated in a small sampling group formed by sera from Brazilians (n = 32). In this context, densitometry analysis of bands signaling reactivity toward the chimeric recombinant proteins IBMP-8.1 and/or – 8.4 led to excellent results (100.0% for both parameters) [75]. Apart from the small quantity of samples tested, the study also portraits an analysis assessment opposite to reality in point-of-care settings and field study. In addition, there are no surveys done with the final formulation. Finally, we emphasize that TR Chagas is currently only at disposal of Brazilian Ministry of Health.

5. Concluding remarks

Many rapid tests were elaborated and evaluated for the detection of *T. cruzi* infection, however, only a few are commercially available. This is particularly worrisome for those populations with poor performance results, such the Mexicans. Conversely to some authors' assertion, these data clearly demonstrate that is still a general demand for improvements (notably assays with higher sensitivity) and development of rapid tests with different antigenic preparations to enhance populational cover with different origins. Furthermore, more studies are required to evaluate if the outperformance detected for two rapid tests is restricted to one ELISA kit or if other immunoassays taken as reference may lead to rapid testing underestimated data. Attending these needs will probably trend an increase of rapid tests use in the frontline diagnosis algorithm given its advantages in both clinical and field practices. In sum, validated rapid testing campaigns and seroprevalence studies have a major role in identifying the areas that require more effective public health actions, besides broaden the diagnosis reach, especially regarding those in asymptomatic phase. In clinical practices, its application in points-of-care and emergency services stands out, as in the case of organ transplantation and women at delivery. In view of the higher rate of early CD diagnosis that can be achieved by rapid testing, it may represent a cost-effective approach in the overall socioeconomic gain. We also stress out that the assistance of those patients remotely located would also benefit from an on-site rapid testing that provides a simultaneous detection of disease progression monitoring marker.

Acknowledgements

This work was supported by CNPq, FAPERJ and FIOCRUZ.

Conflict of interest

The authors declare no conflict of interest.

Author details

Marcelle Almeida Caminha, Ana Luiza Barbosa Godart Cavalcante and Rubem Figueiredo Sadok Menna-Barreto*
Oswaldo Cruz Institute-Fiocruz, Rio de Janeiro, Brazil

*Address all correspondence to: rubemsadok@gmail.com

References

[1] Chagas C. Nova tripanozomiase humana: estudos sobre a morfolojia e o ciclo evolutivo do Schizotrypanum cruzi n. gen., n. sp., ajente etiolojico de nova entidade morbida do homem. Memórias do Instituto Oswaldo Cruz. 1909;**1**:60

[2] Shikanai-Yasuda MA, Carvalho NB. Oral transmission of Chagas disease. Clinical Infectious Diseases. 2012;**54**:845-852. DOI: 10.1093/cid/cir956

[3] Silva-dos-Santos D, Barreto-de-Albuquerque J, Guerra B, Moreira OC, Berbert LR, Ramos MT, et al. Unraveling Chagas disease transmission through the oral route: Gateways to *Trypanosoma cruzi* infection and target tissues. PLoS Neglected Tropical Diseases. 2017;**11**:e0005507. DOI: 10.1371/journal.pntd.0005507

[4] Coura JR, Viñas PA, Junqueira AC. Ecoepidemiology, short history and control of Chagas disease in the endemic countries and the new challenge for non-endemic countries. Memórias do Instituto Oswaldo Cruz. 2014;**109**:856-862. DOI: 10.1590/0074-0276140236

[5] Coura JR. The main sceneries of Chagas disease transmission. The vectors, blood and oral transmissions–a comprehensive review. Memórias do Instituto Oswaldo Cruz. 2015;**110**:277-282. DOI: 10.1590/0074-0276140362

[6] Lidani KCF, Andrade FA, Bavia L, Damasceno FS, Beltrame MH, Messias-Reason IJ, et al. Chagas disease: From discovery to a worldwide health problem. Frontiers in Public Health. 2019;**7**:166. DOI: 10.3389/fpubh.2019.00166

[7] Pérez-Molina JA, Molina I. Chagas disease. The Lancet. 2018;**391**:82-94. DOI: 10.1016/S0140-6736(17)31612-4

[8] Lee BY, Bacon KM, Bottazzi ME, Hotez PJ. Global economic burden of Chagas disease: A computational simulation model. The Lancet Infectious Diseases. 2013;**13**:342-348. DOI: 10.1016/S1473-3099(13)70002-1

[9] Abuhab A, Trindade E, Aulicino GB, Fujii S, Bocchi EA, Bacal F. Chagas' cardiomyopathy: The economic burden of an expensive and neglected disease. International Journal of Cardiology. 2013;**168**:2375-2380. DOI: 10.1016/j.ijcard.2013.01.262

[10] Olivera MJ, Buitrago G. Economic costs of Chagas disease in Colombia in 2017: A social perspective. International Journal of Infectious Diseases. 2020;**91**:196-201. DOI: 10.1016/j.ijid.2019.11.022

[11] Dias JCP. Evolution of Chagas disease screening programs and control programs: Historical perspective. Global Heart. 2015;**10**:193-202. DOI: 10.1016/j.gheart.2015.06.003

[12] DNDi. Chagas disease facts 2022 [Internet]. 2022. Available from: https://dndi.org/diseases/chagas/facts/

[13] Iglesias-Rus L, Romay-Barja M, Boquete T, Benito A, Blasco-Hernández T. The role of the first level of health care in the approach to Chagas disease in a non-endemic country. PLoS Neglected Tropical Diseases. 2019;**13**:e0007937. DOI: 10.1371/journal.pntd.0007937

[14] West HM, Milliren CE, Manne-Goehler J, Davis J, Gallegos J, Perez JH, et al. Effect of clinician information sessions on diagnostic testing for Chagas disease. PLoS Neglected Tropical Diseases. 2022;**16**:e0010524. DOI: 10.1371/journal.pntd.0010524

[15] Sales Junior PA, Molina I, Fonseca Murta SM, Sánchez-Montalvá A, Salvador F, Corrêa-Oliveira R, et al. Experimental and clinical treatment of Chagas disease: A review. The American Journal of Tropical Medicine and Hygiene. 2017;**97**:1289-1303. DOI: 10.4269/ajtmh.16-0761

[16] Jackson Y, Wyssa B, Chappuis F. Tolerance to nifurtimox and benznidazole in adult patients with chronic Chagas' disease. Journal of Antimicrobial Chemotherapy. 2020;**75**:690-696. DOI: 10.1093/jac/dkz473

[17] Pino-Marín A, Medina-Rincón GJ, Gallo-Bernal S, Duran-Crane A, Arango Duque ÁI, Rodríguez MJ, et al. Chagas cardiomyopathy: From Romaña sign to heart failure and sudden cardiac death. Pathogens. 2021;**10**:505. DOI: 10.3390/pathogens10050505

[18] PAHO. Guidelines for the Diagnosis and Treatment of Chagas Disease. Washington, D. C.: PAHO; 2019

[19] López-Monteon A, Dumonteil E, Ramos-Ligonio A, López-Monteon A, Dumonteil E, Ramos-Ligonio A. More than a Hundred Years in the Search for an Accurate Diagnosis for Chagas Disease: Current Panorama and Expectations. Rijeka: IntechOpen; 2019. DOI: 10.5772/intechopen.86567

[20] Carlier Y, Altcheh J, Angheben A, Freilij H, Luquetti AO, Schijman AG, et al. Congenital Chagas disease: Updated recommendations for prevention, diagnosis, treatment, and follow-up of newborns and siblings, girls, women of childbearing age, and pregnant women. PLoS Neglected Tropical Diseases. 2019;**13**:e0007694. DOI: 10.1371/journal.pntd.0007694

[21] Chippaux J-P, Clavijo ANS, Santalla JA, Postigo JR, Schneider D, Brutus L. Antibody drop in newborns congenitally infected by *Trypanosoma cruzi* treated with benznidazole. Tropical Medicine & International Health. 2010;**15**:87-93. DOI: 10.1111/j.1365-3156.2009.02431.x

[22] Ruiz-Lancheros E, Chatelain E, Ndao M. Chagas disease treatment efficacy biomarkers: Myths and realities. In: Altcheh JM, Freilij H, editors. Chagas Disease: A Clinical Approach. Cham: Springer International Publishing; 2019. pp. 323-349. DOI: 10.1007/978-3-030-00054-7_16

[23] Santos FLN, de Souza WV, da Barros MS, Nakazawa M, Krieger MA, de Gomes YM. Chronic Chagas disease diagnosis: A comparative performance of commercial enzyme immunoassay tests. The American Journal of Tropical Medicine and Hygiene. 2016;**94**:1034-1039. DOI: 10.4269/ajtmh.15-0820

[24] Zingales B, Miles MA, Campbell DA, Tibayrenc M, Macedo AM, Teixeira MMG, et al. The revised *Trypanosoma cruzi* subspecific nomenclature: Rationale, epidemiological relevance and research applications. Infection, Genetics and Evolution. 2012;**12**:240-253. DOI: 10.1016/j.meegid.2011.12.009

[25] Magalhães LMD, Gollob KJ, Zingales B, Dutra WO. Pathogen diversity, immunity, and the fate of infections: Lessons learned from *Trypanosoma cruzi* human–host interactions. The Lancet Microbe. 2022;**3**(9):E711-E722. DOI: 10.1016/S2666-5247(21)00265-2

[26] Zingales B. *Trypanosoma cruzi* genetic diversity: Something new for something known about Chagas disease manifestations, serodiagnosis and drug sensitivity. Acta Tropica. 2018;**184**:38-52. DOI: 10.1016/j.actatropica.2017.09.017

[27] Balouz V, Agüero F, Buscaglia CA. Chagas disease diagnostic applications: Present knowledge and future steps. Advances in Parasitology. 2017;**97**:1-45. DOI: 10.1016/bs.apar.2016.10.001

[28] Lozano D, Rojas L, Méndez S, Casellas A, Sanz S, Ortiz L, et al. Use of rapid diagnostic tests (RDTs) for conclusive diagnosis of chronic Chagas disease – field implementation in the Bolivian Chaco region. PLoS Neglected Tropical Diseases. 2019;**13**:e0007877. DOI: 10.1371/journal.pntd.0007877

[29] Médecins Sans Frontières. International meeting: New diagnostic tests are urgently needed to treat patients with Chagas disease. Revista da Sociedade Brasileira de Medicina Tropical. 2008;**41**:315-319. DOI: 10.1590/S0037-86822008000300020

[30] Anfossi L. Rapid Test - Advances in Design, Format and Diagnostic Applications. Ed.; London, UK: IntechOpen; 2018. DOI: 10.5772/intechopen.70916

[31] Egüez KE, Alonso-Padilla J, Terán C, Chipana Z, García W, Torrico F, et al. Rapid diagnostic tests duo as alternative to conventional serological assays for conclusive Chagas disease diagnosis. PLoS Neglected Tropical Diseases. 2017;**11**:e0005501. DOI: 10.1371/journal.pntd.0005501

[32] Roddy P, Goiri J, Flevaud L, Palma PP, Morote S, Lima N, et al. Field evaluation of a rapid immunochromatographic assay for detection of *Trypanosoma cruzi* infection by use of whole blood. Journal of Clinical Microbiology. 2008;**46**:2022-2027. DOI: 10.1128/JCM.02303-07

[33] Chippaux J-P, Santalla JA, Postigo JR, Romero M, Salas Clavijo NA, Schneider D, et al. Sensitivity and specificity of Chagas Stat-Pak test in Bolivia. Tropical Medicine & International Health. 2009;**14**:732-735. DOI: 10.1111/j.1365-3156.2009.02288.x

[34] Castro-Sesquen YE, Saldaña A, Patino Nava D, Paulette Evans D, Bayangos T, DeToy K, et al. Evaluation of 2 lateral flow rapid tests in the diagnosis of Chagas Disease in the Washington Metropolitan Area. Open Forum Infectious Diseases. 2021;**8**:ofab096. DOI: 10.1093/ofid/ofab096

[35] Suescún-Carrero SH, Salamanca-Cardozo LP, Pinazo M-J, Armadans-Gil L. Sensitivity and specificity of two rapid tests for the diagnosis of infection by *Trypanosoma cruzi* in a Colombian population. PLoS Neglected Tropical Diseases. 2021;**15**:e0009483. DOI: 10.1371/journal.pntd.0009483

[36] Mendicino D, Colussi C, Moretti E. Simultaneous use of two rapid diagnostic tests for the diagnosis of Chagas disease. Tropical Doctor. 2019;**49**:23-26. DOI: 10.1177/0049475518813792

[37] Lopez-Albizu C, Danesi E, Piorno P, Fernandez M, García Campos F, Scollo K, et al. Rapid diagnostic tests for *Trypanosoma cruzi* infection: Field evaluation of two registered kits in a region of endemicity and a region of nonendemicity in Argentina. Journal of Clinical Microbiology. 2020;**58**:e01140-20. DOI: 10.1128/JCM.01140-20

[38] Spinicci M, Fumagalli C, Maurizi N, Guglielmi E, Roselli M, Gamboa H, et al. Feasibility of a combined mobile-health electrocardiographic and rapid diagnostic test screening for chagas-related cardiac alterations. Microorganisms. 2021;**9**:1889. DOI: 10.3390/microorganisms9091889

[39] Pinho RT, Waghabi MC, Cardillo F, Mengel J, Antas PR. Scrutinizing the

biomarkers for the neglected Chagas disease: How remarkable! Frontiers in Immunology. 2016;7:306. DOI: 10.3389/fimmu.2016.00306

[40] Chatelain E. Chagas disease research and development: Is there light at the end of the tunnel? Computational and Structural Biotechnology Journal. 2017;**15**:98-103. DOI: 10.1016/j.csbj.2016.12.002

[41] Requena-Méndez A, López MC, Angheben A, Izquierdo L, Ribeiro I, Pinazo MJ, et al. Evaluating Chagas disease progression and cure through blood-derived biomarkers: A systematic review. Expert Review of Anti-Infective Therapy. 2013;**11**:957-976. DOI: 10.1586/14787210.2013.824718

[42] Caminha MA, de Lorena VMB, de Oliveira JW, Perales J, Carvalho PC, Lima DB, et al. *Trypanosoma cruzi* immunoproteome: Calpain-like CAP5.5 differentially detected throughout distinct stages of human Chagas disease cardiomyopathy. Journal of Proteomics. 2019;**194**:179-190. DOI: 10.1016/j.jprot.2018.11.019

[43] Rabelo MMN, Larocca TF, Macêdo CT, Torreão JA, de Souza BSF, Vasconcelos JF, et al. Evaluation of Galectin-3 as a Novel Biomarker for Chagas Cardiomyopathy. 2017;**136**(1):33-39. DOI: 10.1159/000447529

[44] Buekens P, Cafferata ML, Alger J, Althabe F, Belizán JM, Bustamante N, et al. Congenital transmission of *Trypanosoma cruzi* in Argentina, Honduras, and Mexico: An observational prospective study. The American Journal of Tropical Medicine and Hygiene. 2018;**98**:478-485. DOI: 10.4269/ajtmh.17-0516

[45] Truyens C, Dumonteil E, Alger J, Cafferata ML, Ciganda A, Gibbons L, et al. Geographic variations in test reactivity for the serological diagnosis of *Trypanosoma cruzi* infection. Journal of Clinical Microbiology. 2021;**59**:e0106221. DOI: 10.1128/JCM.01062-21

[46] Gamboa-León R, Gonzalez-Ramirez C, Padilla-Raygoza N, Sosa-Estani S, Caamal-Kantun A, Buekens P, et al. Do commercial serologic tests for *Trypanosoma cruzi* infection detect Mexican strains in women and newborns? The Journal of Parasitology. 2011;**97**:338-343. DOI: 10.1645/GE-2545.1

[47] Bern C, Verastegui M, Gilman RH, LaFuente C, Galdos-Cardenas G, Calderon M, et al. Congenital *Trypanosoma cruzi* transmission in Santa Cruz, Bolivia. Clinical Infectious Diseases. 2009;**49**:1667-1674. DOI: 10.1086/648070

[48] Messenger LA, Gilman RH, Verastegui M, Galdos-Cardenas G, Sanchez G, Valencia E, et al. Toward improving early diagnosis of congenital Chagas disease in an endemic setting. Clinical Infectious Diseases. 2017;**65**:268-275. DOI: 10.1093/cid/cix277

[49] Jackson Y, Chatelain E, Mauris A, Holst M, Miao Q, Chappuis F, et al. Serological and parasitological response in chronic Chagas patients 3 years after nifurtimox treatment. BMC Infectious Diseases. 2013;**13**:85. DOI: 10.1186/1471-2334-13-85

[50] Chappuis F, Mauris A, Holst M, Albajar-Vinas P, Jannin J, Luquetti AO, et al. Validation of a rapid immunochromatographic assay for diagnosis of *Trypanosoma cruzi* infection among Latin-American migrants in Geneva, Switzerland. Journal of Clinical Microbiology. 2010;**48**:2948-2952. DOI: 10.1128/JCM.00774-10

[51] Pane S, Giancola ML, Piselli P, Corpolongo A, Repetto E, Bellagamba R,

et al. Serological evaluation for Chagas disease in migrants from Latin American countries resident in Rome, Italy. BMC Infectious Diseases. 2018;**18**:212. DOI: 10.1186/s12879-018-3118-5

[52] Llenas-García J, Hernando A, Fiorante S, Maseda D, Matarranz M, Salto E, et al. Chagas disease screening among HIV-positive Latin American immigrants: An emerging problem. European Journal of Clinical Microbiology & Infectious Diseases. 2012;**31**:1991-1997. DOI: 10.1007/s10096-011-1531-4

[53] Luquetti AO, Ponce C, Ponce E, Esfandiari J, Schijman A, Revollo S, et al. Chagas' disease diagnosis: A multicentric evaluation of Chagas Stat-Pak, a rapid immunochromatographic assay with recombinant proteins of *Trypanosoma cruzi*. Diagnostic Microbiology and Infectious Disease. 2003;**46**:265-271. DOI: 10.1016/s0732-8893(03)00051-8

[54] Ponce C, Ponce E, Vinelli E, Montoya A, de Aguilar V, Gonzalez A, et al. Validation of a rapid and reliable test for diagnosis of Chagas' disease by detection of *Trypanosoma cruzi*-specific antibodies in blood of donors and patients in Central America. Journal of Clinical Microbiology. 2005;**43**:5065-5068. DOI: 10.1128/JCM.43.10.5065-5068.2005

[55] Gruber A, Zingales B. *Trypanosoma cruzi*: Characterization of two recombinant antigens with potential application in the diagnosis of Chagas' disease. Experimental Parasitology. 1993;**76**:1-12. DOI: 10.1006/expr.1993.1001

[56] Sánchez-Camargo CL, Albajar-Viñas P, Wilkins PP, Nieto J, Leiby DA, Paris L, et al. Comparative evaluation of 11 commercialized rapid diagnostic tests for detecting *Trypanosoma cruzi* antibodies in serum banks in areas of endemicity and nonendemicity. Journal of Clinical Microbiology. 2014;**52**:2506-2512. DOI: 10.1128/JCM.00144-14

[57] Da Costa-Demaurex C, Cárdenas MT, Aparicio H, Bodenmann P, Genton B, D'Acremont V. Screening strategy for Chagas disease in a non-endemic country (Switzerland): A prospective evaluation. Swiss Medical Weekly. 2019;**149**:w20050. DOI: 10.4414/smw.2019.20050

[58] Houghton RL, Stevens YY, Hjerrild K, Guderian J, Okamoto M, Kabir M, et al. Lateral flow immunoassay for diagnosis of *Trypanosoma cruzi* infection with high correlation to the radioimmunoprecipitation assay. Clinical and Vaccine Immunology. 2009;**16**:515-520. DOI: 10.1128/CVI.00383-08

[59] InBios. Trypanosoma detect rapid test [Internet]. 2023. Available from: https://inbios.com/trypanosoma-detecttm-rapid-test-intl/

[60] Shah V, Ferrufino L, Gilman RH, Ramirez M, Saenza E, Malaga E, et al. Field evaluation of the InBios Chagas detect plus rapid test in serum and whole-blood specimens in Bolivia. Clinical and Vaccine Immunology. 2014;**21**:1645-1649. DOI: 10.1128/CVI.00609-14

[61] InBios. Chagas detect Plus rapid test [Internet]. 2023. Available from: https://inbios.com/chagas-detecttm-plus-rapid-test-intl-fda-cleared/

[62] Reithinger R, Grijalva MJ, Chiriboga RF, Alarcón de Noya B, Torres JR, Pavia-Ruz N, et al. Rapid detection of *Trypanotsoma cruzi* in human serum by use of an immunochromatographic dipstick test. Journal of Clinical Microbiology. 2010;**48**:3003-3007. DOI: 10.1128/JCM.02474-09

[63] Brutus L, Schneider D, Postigo J, Romero M, Santalla J, Chippaux JP.

Congenital Chagas disease: Diagnostic and clinical aspects in an area without vectorial transmission, Bermejo, Bolivia. Acta Tropica. 2008;**106**:195-199. DOI: 10.1016/j.actatropica.2008.03.009

[64] Silgado A, Gual-Gonzalez L, Sánchez-Montalvá A, Oliveira-Souto I, Goterris L, Serre-Delcor N, et al. Analytical evaluation of dried blood spot and rapid diagnostic test as a new strategy for serological community screening for chronic Chagas disease. Frontiers in Cellular and Infection Microbiology. 2021;**11**:736630. DOI: 10.3389/fcimb.2021.736630

[65] Hopkins T, Gonçalves R, Mamani J, Courtenay O, Bern C. Chagas disease in the Bolivian Chaco: Persistent transmission indicated by childhood seroscreening study. International Journal of Infectious Diseases. 2019;**86**:175-177. DOI: 10.1016/j.ijid.2019.07.020

[66] Whitman JD, Bulman CA, Gunderson EL, Irish AM, Townsend RL, Stramer SL, et al. Chagas disease serological test performance in U.S. blood donor specimens. Journal of Clinical Microbiology. 2019;**57**:e01217-e01219. DOI: 10.1128/JCM.01217-19

[67] Flores-Chavez M, Cruz I, Nieto J, Gárate T, Navarro M, Pérez-Ayala A, et al. Sensitivity and specificity of an operon immunochromatographic test in serum and whole-blood samples for the diagnosis of *Trypanosoma cruzi* infection in Spain, an area of nonendemicity. Clinical and Vaccine Immunology. 2012;**19**:1353-1359. DOI: 10.1128/CVI.00227-12

[68] Flores-Chávez M, Cruz I, Rodríguez M, Nieto J, Franco E, Gárate T, et al. Comparison of conventional and non-conventional serological tests for the diagnosis of imported Chagas disease in Spain. Enfermedades Infecciosas y Microbiología Clínica. 2010;**28**:284-293. DOI: 10.1016/j.eimc.2009.07.005

[69] Roca C, Pinazo MJ, López-Chejade P, Bayó J, Posada E, López-Solana J, et al. Chagas disease among the Latin American adult population attending in a primary care center in Barcelona, Spain. PLoS Neglected Tropical Diseases. 2011;**5**:e1135. DOI: 10.1371/journal.pntd.0001135

[70] Chejade PL, Saumell CR, Posada E, Pinazo MJ, Brustenga JG, Vynieta MP. Utilidad de un test inmunocromatográfico para el cribado de la enfermedad de Chagas en asistencia primaria. Enfermedades Infecciosas y Microbiología Clínica. 2010;**28**:169-171

[71] Navarro M, Perez-Ayala A, Guionnet A, Pérez-Molina JA, Navaza B, Estévez L, et al. Targeted screening and health education for Chagas disease tailored to at-risk migrants in Spain, 2007 to 2010. Eurosurveillance. 2011;**16**(38):19973. DOI: 10.2807/ese.16.38.19973-en

[72] Operon. Simple Chagas WB [Internet]. 2023. Available from: https://operondx.com/wp-content/uploads/pdf/090509_CHAGASWB_web.pdf

[73] Duarte LF, Flórez O, Rincón G, González CI. Comparison of seven diagnostic tests to detect *Trypanosoma cruzi* infection in patients in chronic phase of Chagas disease. Colombia Médica (Cali). 2014;**45**:61-66

[74] Mendicino D, Stafuza M, Colussi C, del Barco M, Streiger M, Moretti E. Diagnostic reliability of an immunochromatographic test for Chagas disease screening at a primary health care centre in a rural endemic area. Memórias do Instituto Oswaldo Cruz. 2014;**109**:984-988. DOI: 10.1590/0074-0276140153

[75] Silva ED, Silva ÂAO, Santos EF, Leony LM, Freitas NEM, Daltro RT, et al. Development of a new lateral flow assay based on IBMP-8.1 and IBMP-8.4 chimeric antigens to diagnose Chagas disease. BioMed Research International. 2020;**2020**:1803515. DOI: 10.1155/2020/1803515

Section 2

Rapid Test in Cancer Diagnostics

Chapter 5

Aptamer Development for Cancer Diagnostic

Fariza Juliana Nordin, Lim Wan Ming, Michelle Yee Mun Teo and Lionel Lian Aun In

Abstract

Early diagnosis improves the prognosis for cancer patients by allowing early intervention to slow or prevent cancer development and lethality. Aptamers are short single-stranded oligonucleotides that have a length of about 25–80 bases. They are produced chemically and extracted using the systematic evolution of ligands by exponential enrichment (SELEX). The use of aptamers as diagnostic tools in cancer is highly recommended due to their ability to recognize various cancer-related molecules and biomarkers with high affinity and specificity. Despite the clear advantages of aptamers, the potential of aptamers in cancer diagnosis is yet to be reached. This chapter will present the best available knowledge on using aptamers as the biorecognition element in the development of cancer biosensors. We will first present the advantages of aptamers in cancer diagnosis as well as various types of SELEX methods with emphasis on clinically relevant samples such as serum, whole cells, and tissue slices. We will also cover the various aptamer detection platforms, such as colorimetric, fluorescence, and electrochemical platforms. Furthermore, the updates on aptamers specific to KRAS mutation detection in cancer will be reviewed. Finally, the future direction of aptamers in cancer diagnosis will also be discussed.

Keywords: aptamer, SELEX, KRAS, cancer, colorectal

1. Introduction

Cancer is a noncommunicable disease that is the second leading cause of death worldwide [1]. Early detection and effective treatment can save life. This is because early detection of cancer is crucial as it allows for timely intervention and treatment before cancer has a chance to metastasize to other parts of the body [2]. Furthermore, it also increased the chances of successful treatment, as the types or mutations of tumors can be screened to determine the most appropriate anticancer drugs for treatment.

Biosensor is a detection device that consists of a biorecognition element for the selective binding of target analytes and a transducer element for converting the binding event to electrical or optical signals (**Figure 1**) [3]. The biorecognition element typically uses biological molecules, such as enzymes, antibodies, or DNA/RNA, for rapid detection of chemicals or biomarkers in various fields such as cancer diagnostic.

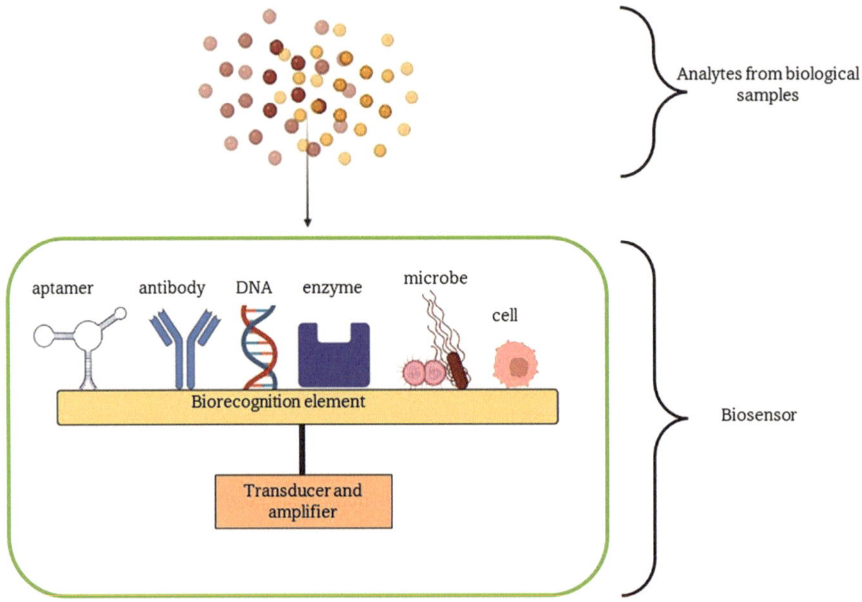

Figure 1.
Biosensor consists of two important parts, which are the biorecognition element and the transducers.

One of the biorecognition elements is aptamers, which are gaining more attention as they can be used to replace antibodies for biomarker discovery and specific diagnostics.

Literally, aptamer means "to fit" (aptus) in Latin. It reflects the important properties of aptamer, which are ability to fold into complex tertiary structures and ability to bind with high affinity [4]. Aptamers are typically single-stranded, 60–100 base pair of nucleic acids has gained tremendous interest as the biorecognition element in the diagnostic tool. There are DNA, RNA, XNA, and peptide aptamers that can be used to detect a wide range of targets. These aptamers differ by the selection process, affinity, and secondary structure formation. DNA aptamer was more preferred because it is more stable due to the C-H bond in the 2′ position of the deoxyribose sugar of the DNA nucleotide [5]. On the other hand, RNA aptamers need stable chemical modification for *in vivo* applications [6]. It is important to incorporate modification during the aptamer selection process to maintain the structure and function of identified aptamers [7].

The main diagnostic figures of merit of aptamer-based approaches are their high sensitivity, specificity, and selectivity. In cancer, the biomarkers are often present at very low concentrations in a highly complex matrix of blood or serum, which can make the diagnosis difficult [8]. Aptamers can overcome the problems as they are able to detect the presence of a target molecule at low concentrations with high accuracy. For example, high levels of cancer biomarker proteins such as prostate-specific antigen (PSA) in blood could indicate prostate cancer. An aptamer-based biosensor developed by Shayesteh et al. was able to detect PSA level as low as 20 pg./mL in human blood serum [9]. Other than that, Xia et al. developed an aptasensor to detect the presence of cancer exosomes with detection limit of 5.2×10^5 particles/mL [10].

The speed and convenience of aptamer-based diagnostic methods are also important figures of merit. Their rapid and convenient methods can be easily performed in a clinical setting with minimal sample preparation and processing, which are

Aptamer	Antibodies
Small (~5–25 kDa)	Relatively big (>125 kDa)
Chemically synthesis *in vitro*	Requires biological systems
Low batch to batch variations	Antibodies activity varies from batch to batch
Low immunogenicity	High immunogenicity
Pharmacokinetics parameters can be changed on demand	Difficult to modify pharmacokinetics parameters
Wide range of targets	Immunogenic molecules
Efficient cellular internalization	Poor internalization into cells
Unlimited shelf life	Limited shelf life
Wide variety of chemical modifications to molecule for diverse functions	Limited modifications to molecule
Sensitive to nuclease degradation	Resistant to nuclease degradation
Very stable	Sensitive to temperature and pH changes

Table 1.
Comparison of aptamer and antibodies.

highly desirable for practical diagnostic applications. Many studies have been done to developed aptasensors that can be used for diagnostic assay in clinical diagnostic laboratories especially those that utilize optical such as colorimetric or fluorescence, and electrochemical sensing platforms [11–14]. Other than that, aptamers are more stable to thermal denaturation when compared to antibodies. It also possesses a longer shelf-life and has no strict requirement for delivery and storage [11].

As summarized in **Table 1**, aptamers can perform beyond what antibodies can offer in diagnostic field. However, the application of aptamer in diagnostic field is still not widely used. This is due to the equipment and processes being uncommon for a clinical laboratory and lack of standardized protocols [15]. Thus, it is important to encourage aptamer-based diagnostic methods that are simple yet rapid and reliable that could be adapted in the point-of-care format for real field applications. This chapter aims to present the best available knowledge on using aptamers as the biorecognition element in the development of cancer biosensors. Different type of SELEX methods used to generate aptamers that target cancer biomarkers in clinically relevant samples such as blood serum, whole cells, and tissue slices was covered. Furthermore, the updates on aptamers specific to KRAS mutation detection in cancer are reviewed.

2. SELEX methodology

Nucleic acid aptamers are derived from the systematic evolution of ligands by exponential enrichment (SELEX) methodology. In this method, an aptamer that has 60–100 nucleotides that can bind specifically to target is isolated from a random library of double-stranded DNA (dsDNA). Then, the dsDNA library is used to synthesize a single-stranded DNA (ssDNA) library or undergoes *in vitro* transcription to produce a ssRNA library [6]. The resulting library sequences can fold and form unique 3D structures. The aptamer unique 3D structure makes them particularly attractive to binding forces such as hydrogen bonds, stacking aromatic

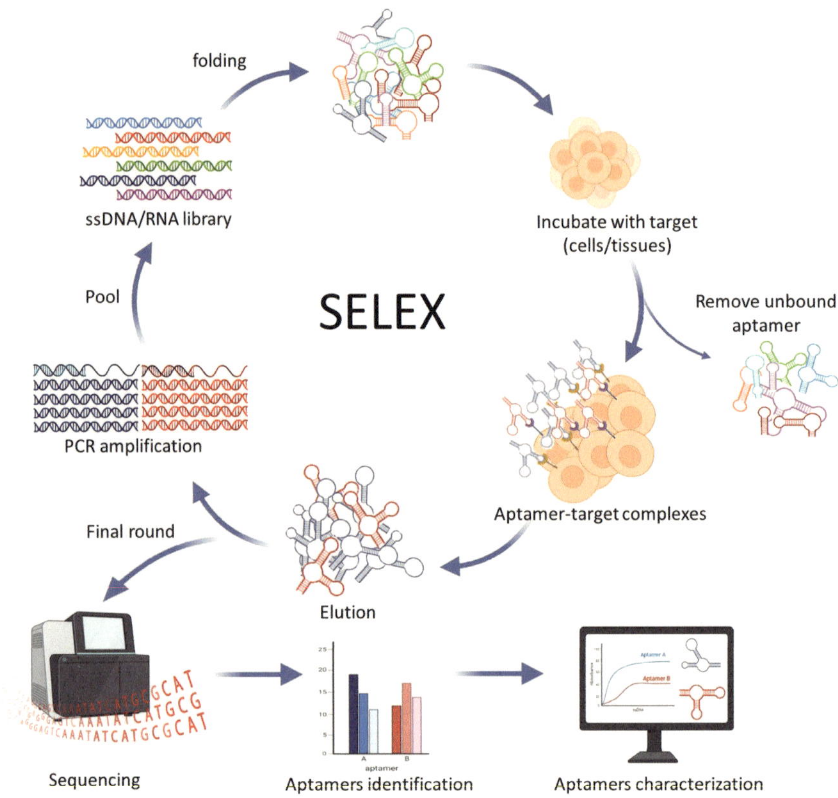

Figure 2.
SELEX process.

rings, salt bridges, Van der Waals forces, various electrostatic interactions, and shape complementary [16]. These different folded oligonucleotide sequences are then incubated with the target of choice. Here, the selection condition, such as temperature, pH, and ionic strength, can be optimized to be compatible with the application of interest [6]. Following that, the oligonucleotides that can bind to the target are retained, while other nonbinding oligonucleotides are washed away. The binding targets are then eluted and amplified using the polymerase chain reaction (PCR) to increase the concentration of the aptamer [17]. The aptamer selection cycle is repeated a few times to improve the aptamer pools that are specific to the target (**Figure 2**).

A variety of SELEX has been developed to obtain aptamers for various targets for cancer diagnosis and treatment (**Table 2**). To name a few, there are cell-SELEX, tissue-SELEX, SOMAmer-SELEX, *in vitro*-SELEX, high-throughput SELEX, capillary electrophoresis SELEX, and magnetic SELEX. However, it is important to develop a medically more relevant aptamer against clinical samples, such as serum, whole cells, and tissue slices. The more commonly used SELEX methods in aptamer-based cancer diagnostic research were cell-SELEX, serum-SELEX, tissue-SELEX, protein-SELEX, and toggle-SELEX. The choice of SELEX procedure is dependent on the specific diagnostic application and the availability of appropriate targets for aptamer selection.

Type of cancer	Aptamer	Type	SELEX	Biomarkers	Ref.
Bladder	EN2-binding ssDNA aptamer	DNA	N/A	Engrailed-2(EN-2)	[18]
	spl3	DNA	Cell-SELEX	Cytoskeleton-associated protein 4 (CKAP4)	[19]
Colorectal	Apta-3, Apta-5	DNA	Protein-SELEX	Carcinoembryonic antigen (CEA) in T84 cells.	[20]
	Seq-2	DNA	Serum-SELEX	N/A	[21]
	ApC1	DNA	Cell-SELEX	Caco-2	[22]
Prostate	A9, A9g, A10, A10-3, A10L, A10-3.2, A10-3-J	RNA	Cell-SELEX	PSMA	[23–26]
	Wy-5a, DML-7, AMH, CSC1, CSC13, E3, PSap4#5,	DNA	Cell-SELEX	Prostate cancer cell lines,	[27–32]
	S3.1/S2.2	DNA	Cell-SELEX	MUC-1 protein	[33]
Gastric	Seq-3, Seq-6, Seq-19, Seq-54	DNA	Serum-SELEX	APOA1, APOA4, PARD2, Importin subunit α-1	[34]
	dual-aptamer (EpCAM and PTK7)-modified immunomagnetic Fe_3O_4 particles (IMNs)	DNA	Cell-SELEX	Circulating tumor cells (CTCs)	[35]
	NCL-Apt-miRNA let-7d chimera	DNA	N/A	Nucleolin	[36]
	PDGC21-T, PDGC21-T-QD	DNA	Cell-SELEX	BGC-823 cells, PDGC tissues	[37]
	cy-apt 20	DNA	Cell-SELEX	AGS cells	[38]
Breast	SE15-8	RNA	*In vitro*-SELEX	ErbB2 protein	[39]
	ex-50.T	RNA	Exo-SELEX	Exosomes	[40]
	CD63-1 and CD63-2	DNA	Competitive-SELEX	CD63 protein	[41]
	sk6Ea	DNA	Cell-SELEX	HER2 protein	[42]
	MF3Ec	DNA	Cell-SELEX	Cell membrane protein PHB2,	[43], [44]
	SKBR3-R1Tr	DNA	3D cell-SELEX	Luminal A breast cancer subtype	[45]
	Apt1, Apt2	DNA	Cell-SELEX Cell-SELEX	SKBR3 cells MDA-MB-231 cells	[46]
Cervical	HPV-07	DNA	SOMAmer-SELEX	Type 16 virus-like-particle (VLP)	[47]
	C-9S	DNA	Cell-SELEX	Ca Ski cells, Hela cells	[48]
Hepatocellular	LY-1, LY-13, LY-46, LY-32, LY-27/45, LY-7/43	DNA	Cell SELEX	HCCLM9 cells	[49]
Various	Ep-DT3-DY647	RNA	*In vitro*-SELEX	Cancer stem cells (CTCs)	[50]
	AS1411	DNA		Nucleolin	[51–54]

Table 2.
Aptamers for cancer.

2.1 Cell-SELEX

In general, cell-SELEX uses intact and living cells as the target to screen a panel of oligonucleotides against multiple cell surface proteins and other macromolecules [55]. The target cells usually were cancer cells, normal cells as contrast cells, or genetically engineered cells that expressed target proteins. This type of SELEX is effective in developing aptamers for cancer biomarker discovery. A major advantage of using cell-SELEX is that the aptamer selection can be performed without prior knowledge of the target protein [56]. Furthermore, aptamers generated using this process can recognize their target in native form as it is not affected by protein purification processes [56]. However, it is important to avoid cell death or remove dead cells population during the selection process. This is because dead cells can cause false positives due to non-specific uptake and binding of oligonucleotides, thus hampered the selection process [56, 57]. High-speed fluorescence activating sorting (FACS) can be used to separate between live and dead or damaged cells [58]. Aptamer selection using this type of SELEX is costly and challenging due to the dynamic and multifaceted structure of the cell membrane as it contains various interacting molecules, such as phospholipids, receptors, transporters, and membrane proteins. Membrane proteins are often embedded within or associated with cell membranes, thus separating aptamers that bind to them can be difficult.

In cell-SELEX method, whole cells are used as targets for aptamers selection. The aptamers selected using this type of SELEX were able to recognize cell surface markers or other cell-associated targets [59]. There were various types of aptamers selected using cell-SELEX that showed the prospects as diagnostics tool in cancer. It has been shown that nucleolin, a cell-surface protein, was often over-expressed in multiple cancer cells [60–62]. Studies showed that AS1411 which is an aptamer selected using cell-SELEX can bind to nucleolin with high affinity [52, 63]. AS1411 was used together with other conjugates for targeted cancer cell imaging. For example, AS1411 aptamer labeled with positron emission tomography (PET) was used as diagnostic imaging agent to detect lung cancer [54]. It can also be conjugated with proteolysis targeting chimeras (PROTAC), gold nanoclusters (GNCs), or carbon dots (CDs) for use in cancer cells targeted imaging [51, 53, 64, 65]. Another study demonstrated that utilizing this aptamer linked with a polymer probe can enable precise and high resolution of nucleolin on the cell surface with selectivity [66].

Prostate-specific membrane antigen (PSMA) is a transmembrane protein, expressed by prostate cancer, hence excellent target for prostate cancer screening [67]. PSMA-specific RNA aptamers, A10 and A9, and DNA PSA-specific aptamer PSap4#5 were the most studied aptamer for prostate cancer diagnosis [68]. A modified version of the A10 aptamer sequence with 2′-fluoro pyrimidine modification that is more stable and less prone to degradation in biological fluid has been developed to make it a potentially more effective diagnostic tool for prostate cancer.

2.2 Tissue-SELEX

Aptamers selected using the tissue-SELEX method could improve target recognition *in vivo* [55]. This method utilizes whole tumor tissue as the target for binding and then isolates aptamers that may bind on different components of the tissues, including extracellular matrix, cellular membranes, and intracellular components [69]. One advantage of using tissue-SELEX to identify aptamers is that the aptamers selected were specific to bind to cancer cells, allowing for their detection and isolation even in heterogeneous population of cells. Li et al. developed DNA aptamer SW1-A that was able to distinguish between liver cancer tissues and normal liver tissues [70]. Other than that, aptamer mcTx-17 was found to be specific to cell membranes of ovarian cancer tissues [71].

2.3 Protein-SELEX

In protein-SELEX, a library of random nucleic acid sequences is incubated with the target protein of interest. The sequences that bind to the protein are then separated from the unbound sequences by using chromatography. In comparison with conventional SELEX, this type of SELEX is utilized for the discovery of novel aptamer for known purified proteins. However, aptamers selected using protein-SELEX may not be able to recognize their corresponding targets *in vitro* especially the large transmembrane molecule in cancer cells [56].

2.4 Serum-SELEX

Serum is a complex mixture of proteins, lipids, hormones, enzymes, electrolytes, and other small molecules. These components can interfere with the detection of cancer biomarkers. Interestingly, aptamers have very high specificity as they can bind to specific epitope on the target molecule, thus lower false-positive rate compared to antibodies, which sometimes can cross-react with similar molecules. In serum-SELEX, the pooled serum is used as target to ensure the diversity of specific target [72]. Negative selection or also known as counter-selection is the initial step that is designed to eliminate sequences that bind to normal serum (**Figure 2**). After exposure to normal serum, the remaining unbound sequences are then carried forward to the next round for positive selection [34]. The unbound sequences are exposed to the target molecule again for further enrichment. Thus, aptamers with improved specificity and selectivity can be obtained for diagnostic application. For example, Apt-5 can bind to human CLEC3b, which plays an important role in infection, inflammation, and tumor immunity [73, 74]. Aptamer Apt-5 can be used as a molecular probe to detect lung cancer. Other than that, a study by Li et al. successfully identified six different aptamers that have high specificity and strong affinity to the sera of lung cancer patients [75]. These aptamers could be further developed as probes for early diagnosis of lung cancer (**Figure 3**).

2.5 Toggle-SELEX

Toggle-SELEX is used to select a species of the cross-reactive aptamer. This type of SELEX is used to generate aptamers that can bind to two different targets. During the selection process, the target molecules are alternated in each round; thus, the selected aptamers can bind both targets most likely to domains conserved between the protein targets. One of the aptamers generated using this type of SELEX was Toggle-25 thrombin aptamer that is used for plasma clot formation and platelet activation [76]. Aptamers generated from toggle-SELEX will facilitate the transition of aptamers from animal models to human subjects.

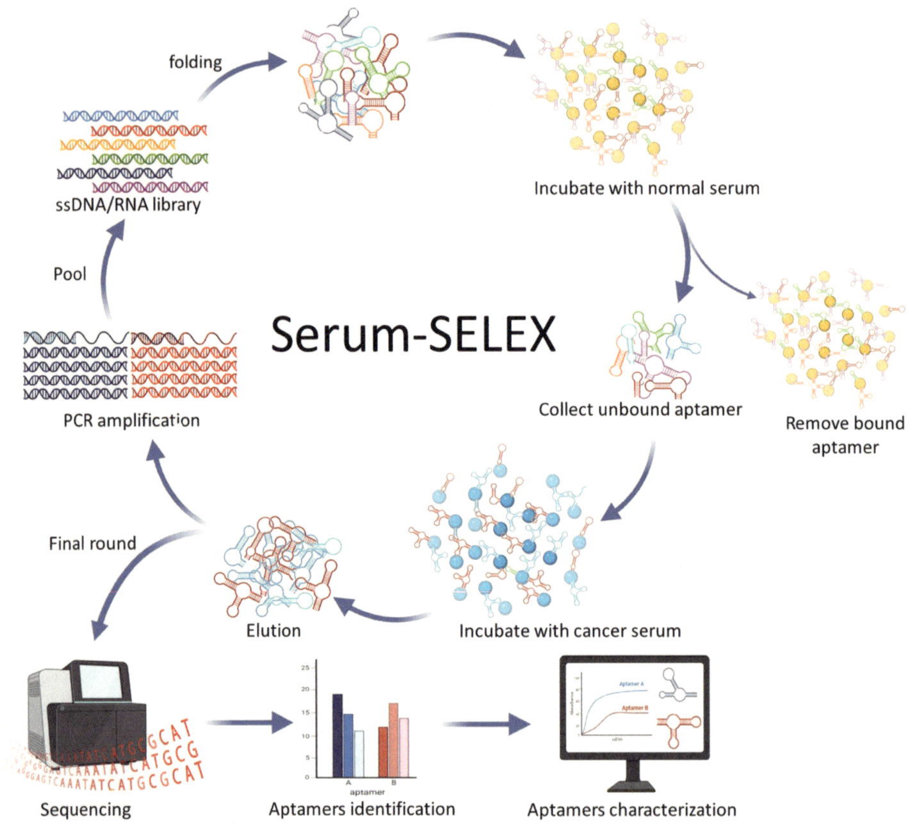

Figure 3.
Serum SELEX.

3. Aptamer for rapid testing and detection platforms

Early detection of cancer often requires the testing of bodily fluids, such as blood, serum or plasma, and tissues. Most of the current design of aptamer-based detection systems often does not account for interfering substances in biological fluids. Using biological fluids such as blood, urine or serum for cancer diagnostic has several challenges. The main reason is a low abundance of cancer biomarkers in blood, making it difficult to detect them using conventional diagnostic assay. This requires the development of highly sensitive and specific assays to accurately detect and quantify cancer biomarkers in blood.

Blood has high nuclease activity; thus, the aptamers must be modified to increase their stability, such as adding sugar, base, or backbone modifications. In addition, the serum is also used for cancer biomarkers detection. However, the components of blood and serum are complex and often difficult to detect low-concentration cancer biomarkers, which hinder early cancer diagnosis. One way to increase the stability and resistance of aptamers against 3′-exonucleases in human serum is by capping the 3′-end with inverted deoxy-thymidine or adding 3′-biotin modification [77]. Studies show that 3′ biotin aptamer modification results in enhanced 3′-nucleases resistance and decrease aptamer clearance from blood circulation *in vivo* [78]. Ni et al. have reviewed other modification steps that can be done to enhance aptamer stability and prolong its half-life [79].

The majority of aptamer-based analytical systems (aptasensors) use optical-based test system that includes colorimetric, fluorescent, and luminescence. Colorimetric aptasensors, such as aptamer-linked immunosorbent assay (ALISA), enzyme-linked oligonucleotide assay (ELONA), or enzyme-linked aptamer assay (ELASA), are dependent on color change of the solution by naked eyes or quantified by using spectrophotometer [80]. Aptamer-based ELISA uses aptamers instead of antibodies to detect the presence of a specific target in a sample. The aptamers can be immobilized on a plate and capture the target, which will be detected using a secondary reagent. Sandwich-type colorimetric aptasensors are known for their high specificity and selectivity, but they typically require the use of aptamer/antibody pairs. Thus, developing completely antibody-free or aptamer/aptamer sandwich-type assays would improve the sensitivity and specificity [11] Other than that, an aptamer can also be immobilized on a test strip and will bind to a specific target such as cancer-related protein in aptamer-based lateral flow assay. This low-cost method has been used to detect various cancer biomarkers such as CD63, CA125, and human osteopontin utilizing nanogold particles as the visualization probe [81–83]. Other than that, the combination of surface-enhanced Raman spectroscopy and lateral flow assay (SERS-LFA) was able to produce convenient, rapid, and sensitive detection of thrombin and platelet-derived growth factor-BB (PDGF-BB) associated with the prostate cancer [84]. Man et al. have developed a chemiluminescence enzyme-linked aptamer assay to simultaneously detect VEGF and CEA cancer biomarkers [85].

Fluorescence-based assays can be used to detect the binding of aptamer to its target molecule by measuring changes in fluorescence polarization or intensity. Labeling the aptamer or target molecules using fluorophores and their signal detection is based on fluorescence resonance energy transfer (FRET), which will reflect the extent of the aptamer-target binding process, thus allowing the quantitative measurement of the target concentration [86]. Several fluorescence biosensors based on aptamers have demonstrated promising results in biological samples such as serum, blood, and urine. Study by Liang et al. showed that aptamers labeled using fluorescence dye and graphene oxide can be used to detect oncoprotein PDGF-BB [87]. In another study, fluorescent probes were used to detect angiogenin in serum samples of healthy and cancer patients [88, 89]. Overall, fluorescence-based assays for aptamer detection can offer real-time monitoring, multiplexing, and nondestructive detection capabilities as reviewed in Ref. [86].

Electrochemical detection platform is based on the measurement of electrical properties such as current or voltage changes due to the binding of an aptamer to its target. The electrode surfaces used in electrochemical aptamer detection include gold electrode [90], carbon electrode [91, 92], and screen-printed electrode [93]. These platforms can support point-of-care testing (POCT) as it allows real-time detection of cancer biomarkers and enables faster diagnosis and treatment [94].

4. Aptamers specific to KRAS mutation

RAS, a guanine nucleotide-binding protein, functions as a transmission of extracellular signals to the interior of the cell. The RAS family is mainly involved in the Ras-Raf-MAPK cell signaling pathway, which plays a key role in cell proliferation, differentiation, and survival [95]. RAS exists in two conformations that can be reversibly switched to an active (guanosine triphosphate [GTP]) or inactive (guanosine diphosphate [GDP]) state through interaction with guanine nucleotide exchange factors or GTPase-activating proteins (GAP). Mutation in RAS causes defective intrinsic GTPase function leading to persistent activations of Ras-Raf-MAPK pathway.

Therefore, RAS superfamily is known as proto-oncogenes, involving Harvey-RAS (HRAS), neuroblastoma-RAS (NRAS), and two splicing variants of Kristen-RAS (KRAS) (KRAS4A and KRAS4B) [96]. About 20% of human tumors are associated with point mutations in the GTPase domain of the RAS gene. Oncogenic NRAS mutations are found in 15–30% of cutaneous malignant melanoma, whereas HRAS mutations are found mostly in oral cavity tumors and hepatocellular carcinomas [97]. To date, oncogenic KRAS mutations are the most frequent and are commonly found in pancreatic (>80%), colorectal (40–50%), and lung (30–50%) carcinomas [98]. Overall, mutations in KRAS genes are necessary for an early event and maintenance of tumorigenesis.

Substitution mutations in the KRAS gene account for 60% of all colorectal cancer cases. Of those, approximately 83% involve codon 12 and 14% involve codon 13, while codon 61 accounts for a minor proportion (2%) [99]. These allelic mutations are located near the GTP binding site, whereby the most clinically frequent substitution from glycine (G) to aspartate (D) was found to occur on codon 12. In primary metastatic colorectal carcinoma, a change in amino acids from glycine (G) to valine (V) at codon 12 occurred more often and this was linked to early mortality. Li et al. suggested that G12D and G12V mutations were independent prognostic factors for poor prognosis in colorectal cancer patients [100]. Similarly, the most frequent substitution of glycine (G) with aspartate (D) in codon 13 has been shown to be associated with the reduced survival rates in colorectal cancer patients [101].

Although RAS isoforms are highly conserved proteins, their carboxy-terminal domain is diverse in terms of structure and posttranslational modifications. After examining the lysine-rich polybasic carboxy-terminal region of KRAS protein, Tanaka and his group were able to identify RNA aptamers that directly target the KRAS4B isotype protein [102]. They applied an improved SELEX method using isothermal RNA amplification to isolated RNA aptamers targeting activated KRAS proteins. A farnesylated peptide model was used to mimic the carboxy-terminal region of KRAS protein for the selection of RNA aptamers against an affinity column. After eluting out the specific binding RNA aptamers from the column, sequences of two binding aptamers were revealed. The binding affinity of these aptamers to the farnesylated peptide is 10-fold stronger than binding to nonfarnesylated peptide indicating these aptamers could recognize the hydrophobic farnesyl moiety of KRAS4B.

In contrast to the discovery of aptamers targeting KRAS4B, C-terminal domain-binding aptamers were unable to distinguish the oncogenic mutant KRAS protein from wild-type KRAS protein. Hence, an RNA aptamer that specifically binds to mutant KRAS protein was engineered using SELEX method [103]. The aptamer selected in this study has a 50-fold greater affinity for mutant KRAS G12V than for wild-type KRAS, whereby KRAS G12V are known to account for 33.6% of total KRAS mutations. In order to study the targets, cDNA-encoding human wild-type KRAS and KRAS G12V proteins were cloned into pET28a(+) expression vector and expressed in *E.coli* BL21. Real-time PCR assessment, surface plasmon resonance analysis, and competitive precipitation experiments were used to confirm the binding specificity and affinity of the RNA aptamer to KRAS protein variants.

5. Conclusion and future direction

Cancer diagnosis often relies on detecting specific biomarkers such as cancer antigens or circulating tumor cells in the serum, cancer tissues, or blood. Aptamers can be designed to bind to these biomarkers and used as the basis for diagnostic tests. They also hold promise as a powerful tool for cancer diagnosis due to their specificity, sensitivity, and versatility. Most cancer biomarkers discovered today are shared among two or more cancer types. Thus, multiplexing of aptamer-based diagnostic assays could greatly improve the accuracy and sensitivity of cancer diagnosis. For colorectal cancer, the search for KRAS mutation variants aptamers is of utmost importance to distinguish patients who will respond to therapy such as epidermal growth factor-based therapy. Incorporation of the existing biosensor device (e.g., glucometer) with the aptamer-based assay could enhance the translation of aptamer-based assay by omitting the design manufacturing and validation of the prototype [80]. Overall, more research is needed to develop clinically relevant aptamers as a diagnostic tool that holds great promise for the future.

Acknowledgements

We would like to thank UCSI University for funding through the Research Excellence and Innovation Grant (REIG-FAS-2022/047).

Conflict of interest

The authors declare no conflict of interest.

Author details

Fariza Juliana Nordin[1,2], Lim Wan Ming[1], Michelle Yee Mun Teo[1] and Lionel Lian Aun In[1*]

1 Faculty of Applied Sciences, UCSI University, Department of Biotechnology, Kuala Lumpur, Malaysia

2 Faculty of Science and Technology, Department of Biological Sciences and Biotechnology, National University of Malaysia, Bangi, Selangor, Malaysia

*Address all correspondence to: lionelin@ucsiuniversity.edu.my

References

[1] Sung H et al. Global cancer statistics 2020: GLOBOCAN estimates of incidence and mortality worldwide for 36 cancers in 185 countries. CA: A Cancer Journal for Clinicians. 2021;**71**(3):209-249

[2] Ginsburg O et al. Breast cancer early detection: A phased approach to implementation. Cancer. 2020;**126**(S10):2379-2393

[3] Kawamura A, Miyata T. Biosensors. In: Ebara M, editor. Biomaterials Nanoarchitectonics. New York: Elsevier; 2016. pp. 157-176

[4] Thiel KW, Giangrande PH. Therapeutic applications of DNA and RNA aptamers. Oligonucleotides. 2009;**19**(3):209-222

[5] Kim DH, Seo JM, Shin KJ, Yang SG. Design and clinical developments of aptamer-drug conjugates for targeted cancer therapy. Biomaterials Research. 2021;**25**(1):42

[6] Odeh F et al. Aptamers chemistry: Chemical modifications and conjugation strategies. Molecules. 2020;**25**(1):3

[7] Kohlberger M, Gadermaier G. SELEX: Critical factors and optimization strategies for successful aptamer selection. Biotechnology and Applied Biochemistry. 2022;**69**(5):1771-1792

[8] Kumar Kulabhusan P, Hussain B, Yüce M. Current perspectives on aptamers as diagnostic tools and therapeutic agents. Pharmaceutics. 2020;**12**(7):646

[9] Shayesteh OH, Ghavami R. A novel label-free colorimetric aptasensor for sensitive determination of PSA biomarker using gold nanoparticles and a cationic polymer in human serum. Spectrochimica Acta. Part A, Molecular and Biomolecular Spectroscopy. 2020;**226**:117644

[10] Xia Y et al. A dual-modal aptasensor based on a multifunctional acridone derivate for exosomes detection. Analytica Chimica Acta. 2022;**1191**:339279

[11] Davydova A, Vorobyeva M. Aptamer-based biosensors for the colorimetric detection of blood biomarkers: Paving the way to clinical laboratory testing. Biomedicine. 2022;**10**(7):1606

[12] Wilkirson EC et al. Affinity-based electrochemical sensors for biomolecular detection in whole blood. Analytical and Bioanalytical Chemistry. 2023;**14**:1-20

[13] Labib M, Sargent EH, Kelley SO. Electrochemical methods for the analysis of clinically relevant biomolecules. Chemical Reviews. 2016;**116**(16):9001-9090

[14] Wang H, Wu T, Li M, Tao Y. Recent advances in nanomaterials for colorimetric cancer detection. Journal of Materials Chemistry B. 2021;**9**(4):921-938

[15] Lakhin AV, Tarantul VZ, Gening LV. Aptamers: Problems, solutions and prospects. Acta Naturae. 2013;**5**(4):34-43

[16] Rahimizadeh K et al. Development of cell-specific aptamers: Recent advances and insight into the selection procedures. Molecules. 2017;**22**(12):2070

[17] Komarova N, Kuznetsov A. Inside the black box: What makes SELEX better? Molecules. 2019;**24**(19):3598

[18] Kim E, Kang M, Ban C. Aptamer-antibody hybrid ELONA that uses hybridization chain reaction to detect a urinary biomarker EN2 for bladder and prostate cancer. Scientific Reports. 2022;**12**(1):11523

[19] Sun X et al. Elucidation of CKAP4-remodeled cell mechanics in driving metastasis of bladder cancer through aptamer-based target discovery. Proceedings of the National Academy of Sciences of The United States of America. 2022;**119**(16):e2110500119

[20] Izabella Abreu, de Melo M, Rodrigues Correa C, da Silva Cunha P, Miranda, de Góes A, Assis Gomes D, Silva, Ribeiro, de Andrade A. DNA aptamers selection for carcinoembryonic antigen (CEA). Bioorganic & Medicinal Chemistry Letters. 2020;**30**(15):127278

[21] Li K et al. Selection and preliminary application of a single stranded DNA aptamer targeting colorectal cancer serum. RSC Advances. 2019;**9**(66):38867-38876

[22] Maimaitiyiming Y, Yang C, Wang Y, Hussain L, Naranmandura H. Selection and characterization of novel DNA aptamer against colorectal carcinoma Caco-2 cells. Biotechnology and Applied Biochemistry. 2019;**66**(3):412-418

[23] Lupold SE. Aptamers and apple pies: A mini-review of PSMA aptamers and lessons from Donald S. Coffey. American Journal of Clinical and Experimental Urology. 2018;**6**(2):78-86

[24] Leach J, Wang A, Ye K, Jin S. A RNA-DNA hybrid aptamer for nanoparticle-based prostate tumor targeted drug delivery. International Journal of Molecular Sciences. 2016;**17**(3):380

[25] Dassie JP et al. Systemic administration of optimized aptamer-siRNA chimeras promotes regression of PSMA-expressing tumors. Nature Biotechnology. 2009;**27**(9):839-846

[26] Rockey WM et al. Rational truncation of an RNA aptamer to prostate-specific membrane antigen using computational structural Modeling. Nucleic Acid Therapeutics. 2011;**21**(5):299-314

[27] Wang Y et al. DNA aptamer evolved by cell-SELEX for recognition of prostate cancer. PLoS One. 2014;**9**(6):e100243

[28] Duan M et al. Selection and characterization of DNA aptamer for metastatic prostate cancer recognition and tissue imaging. Oncotarget. 2016;**7**(24):36436-36446

[29] Kouhpayeh S et al. Antiproliferative effect of a synthetic aptamer mimicking androgen response elements in the LNCaP cell line. Cancer Gene Therapy. 2016;**23**(8):254-257

[30] Wang J et al. Aptamer-conjugated Nanorods for targeted Photothermal therapy of prostate cancer stem cells. Chemistry, an Asian Journal. 2013;**8**(10):2417-2422

[31] Powell Gray B et al. Tunable cytotoxic aptamer–drug conjugates for the treatment of prostate cancer. Proceedings of the National Academy of Sciences. 2018;**115**(18):4761-4766

[32] Savory N, Abe K, Sode K, Ikebukuro K. Selection of DNA aptamer against prostate specific antigen using a genetic algorithm and application to sensing. Biosensors & Bioelectronics. 2010;**26**(4):1386-1391

[33] Crulhas BP, Karpik AE, Delella FK, Castro GR, Pedrosa VA. Electrochemical aptamer-based biosensor developed

to monitor PSA and VEGF released by prostate cancer cells. Analytical and Bioanalytical Chemistry. 2017;**409**(29):6771-6780

[34] Zheng Y et al. DNA aptamers from whole-serum SELEX as new diagnostic agents against gastric cancer. RSC Advances. 2019;**9**(2):950-957

[35] Li C et al. Dual-aptamer-targeted Immunomagnetic nanoparticles to accurately explore the correlations between circulating tumor cells and gastric cancer. ACS Applied Materials & Interfaces. 2022;**14**(6):7646-7658

[36] Ramezanpour M, Daei P, Tabarzad M, Khanaki K, Elmi A, Barati M. Preliminary study on the effect of nucleolin specific aptamer–miRNA let-7d chimera on Janus kinase-2 expression level and activity in gastric cancer (MKN-45) cells. Molecular Biology Reports. 2019;**46**(1):207-215

[37] Li W, Wang S, Zhou L, Cheng Y, Fang J. An ssDNA aptamer selected by cell-SELEX for the targeted imaging of poorly differentiated gastric cancer tissue. Talanta. 2019;**199**:634-642

[38] Cao HY, Yuan AH, Chen W, Shi XS, Miao Y. A DNA aptamer with high affinity and specificity for molecular recognition and targeting therapy of gastric cancer. BMC Cancer. 2014;**14**(1):699

[39] Kim MY, Jeong S. In vitro selection of RNA aptamer and specific targeting of ErbB2 in breast cancer cells. Nucleic Acid Therapeutics. 2011;**21**(3):173-178

[40] Esposito CL et al. Identification of a novel RNA aptamer that selectively targets breast cancer exosomes. Molecular Therapy - Nucleic Acids. 2021;**23**:982-994

[41] Song Z, Mao J, Barrero R, Wang P, Zhang F, Wang T. Development of a CD63 aptamer for efficient cancer immunochemistry and immunoaffinity-based exosome isolation. Molecules. 2020;**25**(23):5585

[42] Liu M et al. An aptamer-based probe for molecular subtyping of breast cancer. Theranostics. 2018;**8**(20):5772-5783

[43] Liu M, Wang Z, Li S, Deng Y, He N. Identification of PHB2 as a potential biomarker of luminal a breast cancer cells using a cell-specific aptamer. ACS Applied Materials & Interfaces. 2022;**14**(46):51593-51601

[44] Liu M et al. Precise discrimination of luminal a breast cancer subtype using an aptamer in vitro and in vivo. Nanoscale. 2020;**12**(38):19689-19701

[45] Nelissen FHT, Peeters WJM, Roelofs TP, Nagelkerke A, Span PN, Heus HA. Improving breast cancer treatment specificity using aptamers obtained by 3D cell-SELEX. Pharmaceuticals. 2021;**14**(4):349

[46] Ferreira D et al. Selection of aptamers against triple negative breast cancer cells using high throughput sequencing. Scientific Reports. 2021;**11**(1):8614

[47] Trausch JJ, Shank-Retzlaff M, Verch T. Development and characterization of an HPV Type-16 specific modified DNA aptamer for the improvement of potency assays. Analytical Chemistry. 2017;**89**(6):3554-3561

[48] Wang J et al. In vitro selection of a DNA aptamer by cell-SELEX as a molecular probe for cervical cancer recognition and imaging. Journal of Molecular Evolution. 2019;**87**(2-3):72-82

[49] Chen H et al. Subtractive cell-SELEX selection of DNA aptamers binding specifically and selectively to hepatocellular carcinoma cells with high metastatic potential. BioMed Research International. 2016;**2016**:5735869

[50] Shigdar S, Lin J, Yu Y, Pastuovic M, Wei M, Duan W. RNA aptamer against a cancer stem cell marker epithelial cell adhesion molecule. Cancer Science. 2011;**102**(5):991-998

[51] Kong T, Zhou R, Zhang Y, Hao L, Cai X, Zhu B. AS1411 aptamer modified carbon dots via polyethylenimine-assisted strategy for efficient targeted cancer cell imaging. Cell Proliferation. 2020;**53**(1):e12713

[52] Jing Y, Cai M, Zhou L, Jiang J, Gao J, Wang H. Aptamer AS1411 utilized for super-resolution imaging of nucleolin. Talanta. 2020;**217**:121037

[53] He S, Gao F, Ma J, Ma H, Dong G, Sheng C. Aptamer-PROTAC conjugates (APCs) for tumor-specific targeting in breast cancer. Angewandte Chemie International Edition in English. 2021;**60**(43):23299-23305

[54] Li J et al. Aptamer imaging with Cu-64 labeled AS1411: Preliminary assessment in lung cancer. Nuclear Medicine and Biology. 2014;**41**(2):179-185

[55] Sola M et al. Aptamers against live targets: Is In vivo SELEX finally coming to the edge? Molecular Therapy. Nucleic Acids. 2020;**21**:192-204

[56] Chen M et al. Development of cell-SELEX technology and its application in cancer diagnosis and therapy. International Journal of Molecular Sciences. 2016;**17**(12):2079

[57] Chen C, Zhou S, Cai Y, Tang F. Nucleic acid aptamer application in diagnosis and therapy of colorectal cancer based on cell-SELEX technology. NPJ Precision Oncology. 2017;**1**(1):37

[58] Germer K, Leonard M, Zhang X. RNA aptamers and their therapeutic and diagnostic applications. International Journal of Biochemistry and Molecular Biology. 2013;**4**(1):27-40

[59] Cibiel A, Dupont DM, Ducongé F. Methods to identify aptamers against cell surface biomarkers. Pharmaceuticals. 2011;**4**(9):1216-1235

[60] Wang Y et al. Nucleolin-targeted extracellular vesicles as a versatile platform for biologics delivery to breast cancer. Theranostics. 2017;7(5):1360-1372

[61] Carvalho LS, Gonçalves N, Fonseca NA, Moreira JN. Cancer stem cells and nucleolin as drivers of carcinogenesis. Pharmaceuticals. 2021;**14**(1):60

[62] Brignole C et al. Cell surface Nucleolin represents a novel cellular target for neuroblastoma therapy. Journal of Experimental & Clinical Cancer Research. 2021;**40**(1):180

[63] Vindigni G et al. AS1411 aptamer linked to DNA nanostructures diverts its traffic inside cancer cells and improves its therapeutic efficacy. Pharmaceutics. 2021;**13**(10):1671

[64] Ghahremani F, Shahbazi-Gahrouei D, Kefayat A, Motaghi H, Mehrgardi MA, Javanmard SH. AS1411 aptamer conjugated gold nanoclusters as a targeted radiosensitizer for megavoltage radiation therapy of 4T1 breast cancer cells. RSC Advances. 2018;**8**(8):4249-4258

[65] Motaghi H, Mehrgardi MA, Bouvet P. Carbon dots-AS1411 aptamer nanoconjugate for ultrasensitive

spectrofluorometric detection of cancer cells. Scientific Reports. 2017;**7**(1):10513

[66] Fabre L et al. Fluorescent polymer-AS1411-aptamer probe for dSTORM super-resolution imaging of endogenous Nucleolin. Biomacromolecules. 2022;**23**(6):2302-2314

[67] Haberkorn U, Eder M, Kopka K, Babich JW, Eisenhut M. New strategies in prostate cancer: Prostate-specific membrane antigen (PSMA) ligands for diagnosis and therapy. Clinical Cancer Research. 2016;**22**(1):9-15

[68] Campos-Fernández E et al. The use of aptamers in prostate cancer: A systematic review of theranostic applications. Clinical Biochemistry. 2021;**93**:9-25

[69] Dua P, Kim S, Lee D. Nucleic acid aptamers targeting cell-surface proteins. Methods. 2011;**54**(2):215-225

[70] Li L et al. Identification of a new DNA aptamer by tissue-SELEX for cancer recognition and imaging. Analytical Chemistry. 2021;**93**(19):7369-7377

[71] Tsai Y-C, Lin C-S, Lin C-N, Hsu K-F, Lee G-B. Screening aptamers targeting the cell membranes of clinical cancer tissues on an integrated microfluidic system. Sensors and Actuators B Chemical. 2021;**330**:129334

[72] Wang T et al. A universal strategy designed for selecting bench-to-bedside aptamers to serum and validated in hepatocellular carcinoma diagnosis. Microchemical Journal. 2019;**150**:104152

[73] Guo Y et al. CLEC3B identified as a potential lung cancer biomarker in serum by aptamer-capture technology. Chemistry Select. 2021;**6**(22):5640-5645

[74] Zhao Y et al. Identification of a novel DNA aptamer that selectively targets lung cancer serum. RSC Advances. 2021;**11**(53):33759-33769

[75] Li K et al. Screening of specific nucleic acid aptamers binding tumor markers in the serum of the lung cancer patients and identification of their activities. Tumor Biology. 2017;**39**(7):101042831771712

[76] White R et al. Generation of species cross-reactive aptamers using 'toggle' SELEX. Molecular Therapy. 2001;**4**(6):567-573

[77] Zhuo Z et al. Recent advances in SELEX technology and aptamer applications in biomedicine. International Journal of Molecular Sciences. 2017;**18**(10):2142

[78] Dougan H, Lyster DM, Vo CV, Stafford A, Weitz JI, Hobbs JB. Extending the lifetime of anticoagulant oligodeoxynucleotide aptamers in blood. Nuclear Medicine and Biology. 2000;**27**(3):289-297

[79] Ni S et al. Recent Progress in aptamer discoveries and modifications for therapeutic applications. ACS Applied Materials & Interfaces. 2021;**13**(8):9500-9519

[80] Sharma TK, Bruno JG, Dhiman A. ABCs of DNA aptamer and related assay development. Biotechnology Advances. 2017;**35**(2):275-301

[81] Yu Q et al. Development of a lateral flow aptamer assay strip for facile identification of theranostic exosomes isolated from human lung carcinoma cells. Analytical Biochemistry. 2020;**594**:113591

[82] Mukama O et al. A highly sensitive and specific lateral flow aptasensor for the detection of human osteopontin. Talanta. 2020;**210**:120624

[83] Tripathi P, Sachan M, Nara S. Novel ssDNA ligand against ovarian cancer biomarker CA125 with promising diagnostic potential. Frontiers in Chemistry. 2020;**8**:400

[84] Cao X, Song Q, Sun Y, Mao Y, Lu W, Li L. A SERS-LFA biosensor combined with aptamer recognition for simultaneous detection of thrombin and PDGF-BB in prostate cancer plasma. Nanotechnology. 2021;**32**(44):445101

[85] Man J et al. Simultaneous detection of VEGF and CEA by time-resolved Chemiluminescence enzyme-linked aptamer assay. International Journal of Nanomedicine. 2020;**15**:9975-9985

[86] Musumeci D, Platella C, Riccardi C, Moccia F, Montesarchio D. Fluorescence sensing using DNA aptamers in cancer research and clinical diagnostics. Cancers (Basel). 2017;**9**(12):174

[87] Liang J, Wei R, He S, Liu Y, Guo L, Li L. A highly sensitive and selective aptasensor based on graphene oxide fluorescence resonance energy transfer for the rapid determination of oncoprotein PDGF-BB. Analyst. 2013;**138**(6):1726

[88] Li W, Yang X, Wang K, Tan W, Li H, Ma C. FRET-based aptamer probe for rapid angiogenin detection. Talanta. 2008;**75**(3):770-774

[89] Li W et al. Real-time imaging of protein internalization using aptamer conjugates. Analytical Chemistry. 2008;**80**(13):5002-5008. DOI: 10.1021/ac800930q

[90] Ilyas A, Asghar W, Allen PB, Duhon H, Ellington AD, Iqbal SM. Electrical detection of cancer biomarker using aptamers with nanogap break-junctions. Nanotechnology. 2012;**23**(27):275502

[91] Yeh F-Y, Liu T-Y, Tseng I-H, Yang C-W, Lu L-C, Lin C-S. Gold nanoparticles conjugates-amplified aptamer immunosensing screen-printed carbon electrode strips for thrombin detection. Biosensors & Bioelectronics. 2014;**61**:336-343

[92] Khoshfetrat SM, Mehrgardi MA. Amplified detection of leukemia cancer cells using an aptamer-conjugated gold-coated magnetic nanoparticles on a nitrogen-doped graphene modified electrode. Bioelectrochemistry. 2017;**114**:24-32

[93] Ferreira DC, Batistuti MR, Bachour B, Mulato M. Aptasensor based on screen-printed electrode for breast cancer detection in undiluted human serum. Bioelectrochemistry. 2021;**137**:107586

[94] Omage JI et al. Cancer diagnostics and early detection using electrochemical Aptasensors. Micromachines (Basel). 2022;**13**(4):522

[95] Fernandez-Medarde A, Santos E. Ras in cancer and developmental diseases. Genes & Cancer. 2011;**2**(3):344-358

[96] Burge RA, Hobbs GA. Not all RAS mutations are equal: A detailed review of the functional diversity of RAS hot spot mutations. Advances in Cancer Research. 2022;**153**:29-61

[97] Kodaz H et al. Frequency of RAS mutations (KRAS, NRAS, HRAS) in human solid cancer. Eurasian Journal of Medicine and Oncology. 2017;**1**(1):1-7

[98] Timar J, Kashofer K. Molecular epidemiology and diagnostics of KRAS mutations in human cancer. Cancer and Metastasis Reviews. 2020;**39**(4):1029-1038

[99] Hobbs GA, Der CJ, Rossman KL. RAS isoforms and mutations in cancer at a glance. Journal of Cell Science. 2016;**129**(7):1287-1292

[100] Li W et al. Not all mutations of KRAS predict poor prognosis in patients with colorectal cancer. International Journal of Clinical and Experimental Pathology. 2019;**12**(3):957-967

[101] Badic B et al. Predictors of survival in elderly patients with metastatic colon cancer: A population-based cohort study. Cancers (Basel). 2022;**14**(21):5208

[102] Tanaka Y, Akagi K, Nakamura Y, Kozu T. RNA aptamers targeting the carboxyl terminus of KRAS Oncoprotein generated by an improved SELEX with isothermal RNA amplification. Oligonucleotides. 2007;**17**(1):12-21

[103] Jeong S, Han SR, Lee YJ, Kim JH, Lee S-W. Identification of RNA aptamer specific to mutant KRAS protein. Oligonucleotides. 2010;**20**(3):155-161

Chapter 6

The Development of Oral Therapeutic Vaccine against Cancer and Working out on the Fast Testing of Immunogenic and Oncolytic Effector Antigens

Natalya Rekoslavskaya, Rurik Salyaev and Alexey Stolbikov

Abstract

In the study of "the herd immunity", it was found that antigenic "late" proteins L1 of human papillomavirus of types 6,16,18,31 and 45, "early" proteins E2, E6 and E7 induced the generation of interferon, CD4/CD8 T lymphocytes and T cell receptors, as well as apoptotic enzymes: granzyme B, perforin and granulysin in mice peripheric mononuclear blood cells and in splenocytes (according to Elispot). Cancer HeLa cells provoked tumour formation in mice testis and in intact lungs in a month after injection and in isolated lungs after 1–2 days of inoculation. "Early" protein E2, L-amino acid oxidase and D-amino acid oxidase blocked the growth of HeLa cells in vitro, working as an effector. There was the activation of the generation of interferon, immunogenic T lymphocytes as well as apoptotic enzymes: granzyme B, perforin and granulysin in blood, spleen and lung T lymphocytes in tumours of isolated lungs mice treated with HeLa cells. Even when anti-PD-L1 antibody ("checkpoint" control receptor for cancer blocking) was added to isolated tumorigenic mice lung, regardless of the presence of HeLa cells, there was the induction of the immunogenicity. The testing of immunogenic and oncolytic activities of antigens via isolated lung tumour formation lasted 5–7 days including Elispot and HeLa inoculation and provided rapid analysis of immunogenic effector activity and tumour suppressors.

Keywords: human papillomavirus (HPV), antigenic "early" and "late" proteins of HPV (6,16,18,31 and 45 types), induction of the generation of interferon, CD4/CD8 T lymphocytes, T cell receptor, regression of mice testis and lung tumours by HPV16 E2, activation of apoptotic enzymes: Granzyme B, perforin and granulysin, immunogenic and oncolytic effector activities of L-amino acid oxidase and D-amino acid oxidase

1. Introduction

Immune surveillance of cancer is very necessary for host surviving in order to escape carcinogenesis [1]. According to data GLOBOCAN (WHO Agency) in

2022 year, there were registered as much as 1,918,030 new cancer cases and 609,360 cancer deaths that means 350–400 deaths cases per day [2].

Cancer in most cases is a comorbidity and mortality incidence together with HIV, hepatitis B and papillomavirus (HPV) diseases because of weakening of the immune system [3, 4]. Even in every cancer overgrowth, there were usually found papillomaviruses.

Therefore there is an urgent need to develop strategy provided common protection from infections and toxins for therapeutic vaccine, that can fully eliminate malignant cells.

In adult humans, the number of T lymphocytes is close to the quantity of $10^{11–15}$ mostly representing naive cells, which means they are uncharged by any epitopes [5, 6]. These naive T cells resident 40% of the spleen, in peripheral blood up to 50%, and the other of all internal organs: lungs, liver, lymphatic organs etc., have their own depot of T cells as well naive to be ready for activating by external stimuli. The life span of different T lymphocytes can be: for effector natural killer cells of the order 8–10 days, for most peripheral T cells can remain in a resting state for a long period (months in rodents and years in humans) [7, 8].

The huge amount of T naive cells allows us to suspect that their turnover is not so long, and nevertheless, the resting (even still huge) amount of T cells needs to be continuously activated by different effectors in order to support the immune system successfully [9].

The aim of a therapeutic vaccine against cancerogenic HPV is to induce in vivo virus-specific T-cell response against established HPV infections and lesions. At the same time, be sure that vaccine-induced T cells can reach the tumour site and perform their functions without limitation.

A range of approaches were undertaken for the creation of therapeutic vaccines against HPVs: increasing CD4/CD8 T cell response, DNA, RNA, attenuated viral and bacterial, peptide-based, protein-based or on the basis of dendritic cells. But no vaccines were licenced for therapeutic use [10].

The most attention attracted the "early" oncogenes: E6 targeting oncosupressor p53 and E7 interacting with pRB and reducing oncogenic strength. But no significant results were achieved [10]. The therapeutic vaccine against recurrent respiratory papillomatoses on the base vaccinia virus MVA with bovine "early" protein E2 BPV completely regressed laryngeal papillomatosis. The immune response was assessed by the increase of CD4/CD8 T lymphocytes [11].

In order to develop the oral therapeutic vaccine, the aim of our work was to elaborate on the rapid screening system of antigens in order to evaluate their immunogenic and oncolytic specificities and activities. For this purpose, antigenic proteins of papillomaviruses of high-risk oncogenes types of HPV16, 18, 31, 45 and unrelated anogenital type of HPV6 of major coat protein L1 of the "late" expression of the viruses (**Figure 1**) were employed. The regulatory protein of "early" expression of HPV16 E2, well known as tumour supersupressor, was recruited to study its immunogenic and oncolytic activities for the perspectives of the development of a therapeutic vaccine against cancer.

The fast-growing tumours perhaps revealed a rapid protein/amino acid turnover, so the L-amino acid oxidase (LAAO) and D-amino acid oxidase (DAAO) were chosen to study their participation in tumour regression.

DOI: http://dx.doi.org/10.5772/intechopen.1001912

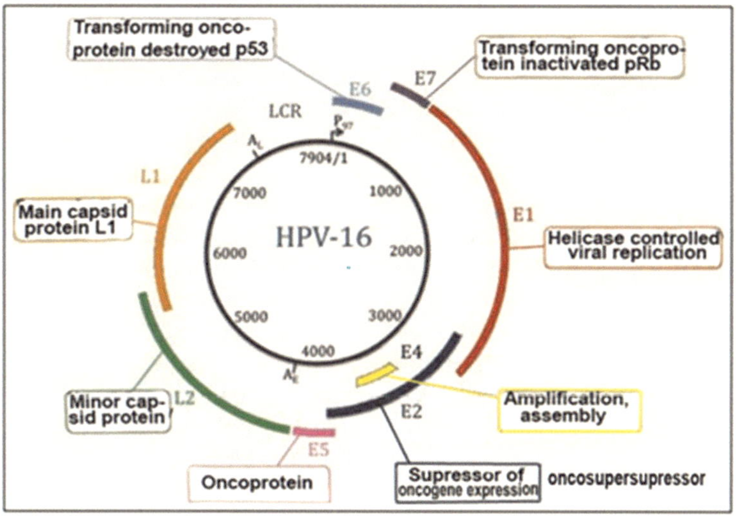

Figure 1.
Physical map of high-risk oncogenic virus HPV16.

2. Methodology

2.1 The genetic constructs and synthetic capacity of the plant virus expression system on the basis of tomato fruit

To synthesise antigenic proteins of HPV6 L1, HPV16, 18, 31 and 45 L1, HPV16 E2, our own author genetic constructs were designed in which RNA-dependent RNA-polymerase (RdRP from Cucumber mosaic virus) played the pivotal role [12]. According to our design, a company Genscript (USA), synthesised eight genetic constructs for the development of prophylactic and therapeutic vaccines against HPV viruses for the production of target proteins in plant viral expression system on the basis of tomato fruit (**Figure 2**).

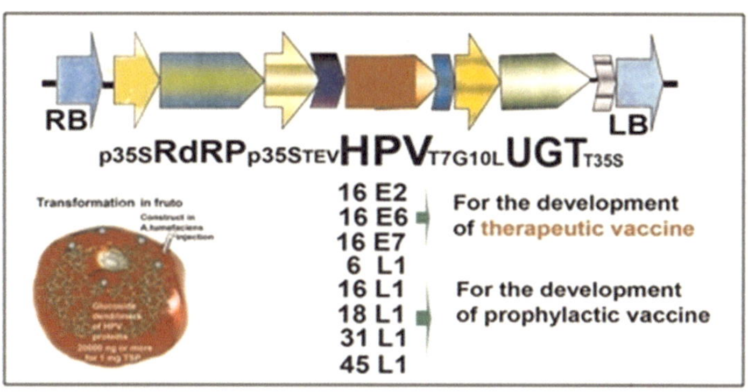

Figure 2.
The plant viral expression system for the production of target antigenic HPV proteins on the basis of tomato fruit.

2.2 Qualitative and quantitative analyses

SDS electrophoresis has been done in Phastsystem apparatus with appropriate buffer strips and ready-to-use plates with PAAG gradient of 8–15% (Amersham, UK). The programme attached to the device was №3 for protein separation [12–14].

The quantities of antigenic proteins synthesised in tomato were estimated by ELISA with appropriate target standard of commercial papillomavirus proteins from companies Santa Cruz Biotech. Inc. and Genway Biotechnology Inc. (USA) [12, 13]. Commercial primary and secondary antibodies of the same companies were used in ELISA.

For Elispot analyses, peripheral mononuclear blood cells (PMBC), splenocytes and T lymphocytes from mice lungs were used. For the isolation of T lymphocytes, fresh or stored at −62°C, blood samples were centrifuge for the flotation at 700 g for 7 min at 4°C. To isolate T lymphocytes from spleen or lungs, their tissues were cut for very many tiny pieces with the needle from steryl syringe in 1 ml of DMEM. The fractions of T lymphocytes were purified by flotation at 700 g in refrigerator centrifuge for 7 min. The fractions were checked in microscope.

These preparations were used in Elispot analyses with antibodies of a company Abcam recruiting HPV16 E2, LAAO or DAAO as activators (effectors). To study the activation of immune system, Elispot analysis was provided with antibodies from the company Abcam (UK) as follows: murine IFNγ ELISPOT KIT [AB64029], rabbit monoclonal [EPR1108] to interferon-gamma (AB133566), Anti-T-Cell Receptor antibody (JOVI.1) (AB5465) mouse monoclonal, rabbit monoclonal Anti-CD4 antibody [EPR19514] (AB183685), rabbit monoclonal Anti-CD8 alpha (SP16) antibody [EPR21769] (AB217344) [14–17], rabbit monoclonal antibodies for enzymes of apoptosis: rabbit polyclonal Anti-Granzyme B (AB53097), rat monoclonal Anti-Perforin antibody [CB5.4] (AB16074), Anti-Human Granulysin (AB213787) monoclonal. Second antibody were goat immunoglobulins to mice conjugated with alkaline phosphatase and substrates BCIP/NBT (5-bromo-4-chloro-3-indolylphosphate/ nitrotetrazolium blue (Sigma, USA).Anti-PD-1 Antibody Clone G4 MABC1132-100UG, monoclonal, from hamster (Armenian) Sigma-Aldrich, USA) and Anti-PDL1M1/CLP36 antibody [EPR7186] ab129015 rabbit monoclonal were used in the experiments to control "check-point" receptors in mice lung tumours.

2.3 The description of experiments with mice

Mice were grown in vivarium with standard conditions. All necessary activities for their maintenance were completed. For experiments, baby mice were selected and grown up in the same cage in order to escape differences in keeping.

HeLa cells were purchased from the company "Biolot" (Saint Petersburg, Russia Federation) and were grown in Corning flasks in DMEM with 10% of bovine fetal serum. Before experiments, HeLa cells were kept at −62°C in DMEM+bovine fetal serum with the addition of 30% of glycerine for cryoconservation. The viability of HeLa cells was detected with trypan blue dye colouring dead cells in dark blue colour. For the injection of mice, HeLa cells were grown in flasks until monolayer of cells covered the bottom of the flasks. The 100 μl of suspension of HeLa cells was injected into the hips of mice with syringe, and the maintenance of animals was as before.

Mice orally vaccinated at the age of 6 months with 500 mg of HPV16 E2 from tomato vaccine material three times with the interval of 1 month. Collected samples of peripheral blood were stored at -62°C before analyses.

In some experiments, injected mice were orally vaccinated after one month, and after 1 month of the last vaccination, they were used for blood sampling and the isolation of lungs and spleen.

For histological analyses and to study the cell state in lung tumours that appeared after the inoculation of lungs with cancer HeLa cells and after vaccination, the microtome slices of these lung tumours were prepared via classical section waxing techniques and staining with haematoxylin by Carazzi. A light microscope with magnification x 360–900 was equipped with a video camera with programme C310 NG Levenhuk (USA) with a resolution of 2048–1536 pc.

3. Results. The study of immunogenic activities of antigenic prophylactic and therapeutic proteins

3.1 The possibility of using prophylacic vaccines as therapeutics

Our plant viral expression system, according to design, produced as much as 25–30 μg of the corresponding antigenic protein per 1 mg of total soluble protein (TSP) [12]. Only one appropriate band was found after electrophoresis without any other impurities in the field that allowed the use of crude buffer extracts of transgenic tomato fruit to escape any multistep and cost purification (**Figure 3**) [12 14].

All these antigenic proteins synthesised in tomato fruit were used for the induction of antibody synthesis in peripheral blood of mice (**Figure 4**).

Mice blood serum samples are the excellent model to study the antibody development and the immune system activation upon oral vaccination. Antibodies raised in mice in our experiments (**Figure 4**) have strong avidity, very high titre and broad specificity to different types of antigens of HPV L1. According to bioinformatic

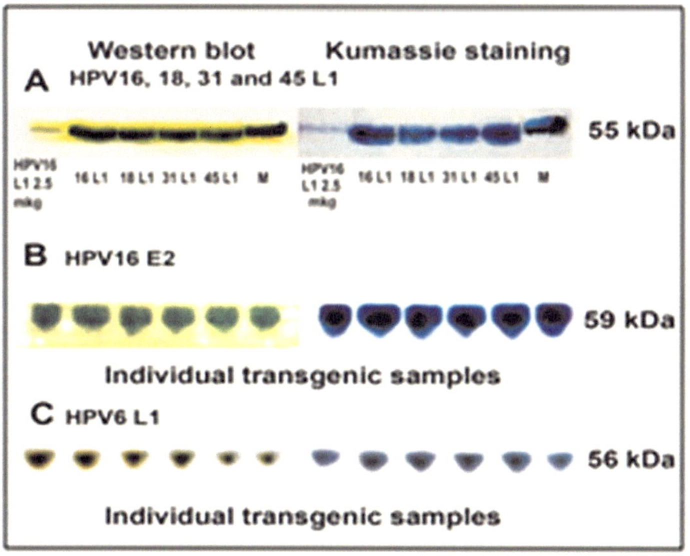

Figure 3.
The electrophoresis and western blot of crude buffer extracts with antigenic proteins: A - HPV16, 18, 31, 45 L1; B - HPV16 E2; C - HPV6 L1 synthesised in plant viral expression system on the basis of tomato fruit. Standard - 2.5 μg of HPV16 L1 (Santa Cruz biotech., USA).

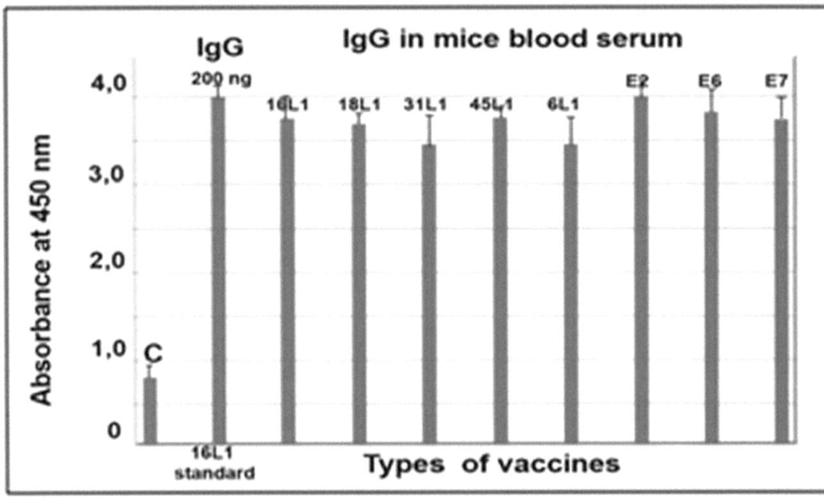

Figure 4.
Antibodies to different types of antigenic proteins of HPV developed in mice blood serum after oral vaccination of mice with appropriate oral vaccines. 200 ng HPV16 L1 is a standard from company Santa Cruz biotech (USA). C-serum from control unvaccinated mice.

analyses (gathered from database SYFPEITHI), there are common epitops (decamers) in all proteins sequences of HPV L1 (means related to one family of 16, 18, 31, 45 L1 types and unrelated from noncarcinogenous anogenital 6 L1 type) but not to HPV16 E2 or LAAO or DAAO of protein sequences (**Table 1**).

Antigenic protein from unrelated noncarcinogenous anogenital type HPV6 L1 was able to be highly active in the induction of the synthesis of interferon (INF), CD4/CD8 ligands of T lymphocytes from peripheral mononuclear blood cells (PMBC) of mice orally vaccinated with tomato vaccine material transgenic with HPV16, 18, 31 and 45 L1 types (**Figure 5**) (**Table A1**) [14].

(Here and further the numbers of coloured immunospots were presented in the Tables in Supplement).

Due to the fact that antigenic coat protein L1 of types HPV16, 18, 31 and 45 usually used for the development of prophylactic vaccines like Gardasil or Cervarics but not for the therapeutical vaccines, was able to induce immune response, it might be consumed that there was a block step on the way lying of above mentioned antigenic proteins L1 to the direction provided the regression of tumours.

Conversely, there is no need to create multivalented prophylactic vaccines like 9-Gardasil if a great immune response is possibly provided by few antigenic proteins of high immunogenic activity.

Nevertheless, it cannot be excluded that the therapeutical potential of prophylactic vaccines should be investigated and improved using several approaches.

3.2 The experimental induction of carcinogenesis by HeLa cells injected in mice

To evoke carcinogenesis, the injection of 100 μl of suspension of cancer HeLa cells was done into the hip muscle of male or female mice, and after 1 month of the inoculation, different tumours were observed outside and inside of mice bodies (**Figure 6**).

Type of HPV	Position	Peptide
HPV16 L1	**12**	**YLPPVPVSKV**
	304	*AQIFNKPYWL
	372	**LQFIFQLCKI**
HPV18 L1	181	SQGDCPPLEL
	12	**YLPPPSVARV**
	304	**SQLFNKPYWL**
HPV31 L1	**12**	**YLPPVPVSKV**
	69	LQYRVFRVRL
	373	LQFIFQLCKI
HPV45 L1	**12**	**YLPPPSVARV**
	307	SQLFNKPYWL
	464	DQYPLGRKFL
HPV6 L1	86	SLFDPTTQRL
	300	AQLFNKPYWL
	101	GLEVGRGQPL
HPV16 E2	199 79 350	GQVILCPTSV LQAIELQPTL WQRDQFLSQV
L-amino acid oxidase [from Crotalus adamanteus] LAAO	271 426 171	VQVHFNARVI IQTFCHPSMI QLYVESLRKV
D-amino acid oxidase [from pig kidney] DAAO	203 97 296	LLQPGRGQII GLTPVSGYNL PQVRLEREQL

**Similar epitops (decamers) are coloured in blue and yellow.*

Table 1.
Predicted antigenic determinants for T cells (HLA-B13 decamers) according to database SYFPEITHI.

To induce the regression of the testis tumours, the antigenic oncosupersupressive protein HPV16 E2 was employed. As can be observed in **Figure 7**, testis tumours appeared 1 month after the injection of mice with cancer cells HeLa. With these tumours male mice stayed still alive and survived during another half a year. Upon ELISA and Elispot analyses, there was registered a significant increase in the content of interferon (INF) and in the amount of generations of CD4/CD8 T lymphocytes in PMBC and in splenocytes (**Figure 8**). After the vaccination with HPV16 E2 (500 mg per mouse), in 2 days, testis tumours became smaller and later disappeared after 1–2 months [15].

The content of newly synthesised INF in PMBC and splenocytes was close to 62 ng per well of the microplate in ELISA analysis. In addition, the contents of CD4/CD8 T lymphocytes increased after vaccination as well were significantly high (**Figure 9**).

During the investigation of internal tumours that appeared in mice bodies after the injection with cancer HeLa cells, it was found that mice lungs were very sensitive and began to proliferate in the next few days with tumours formation of different sizes and types (**Figure 10**).

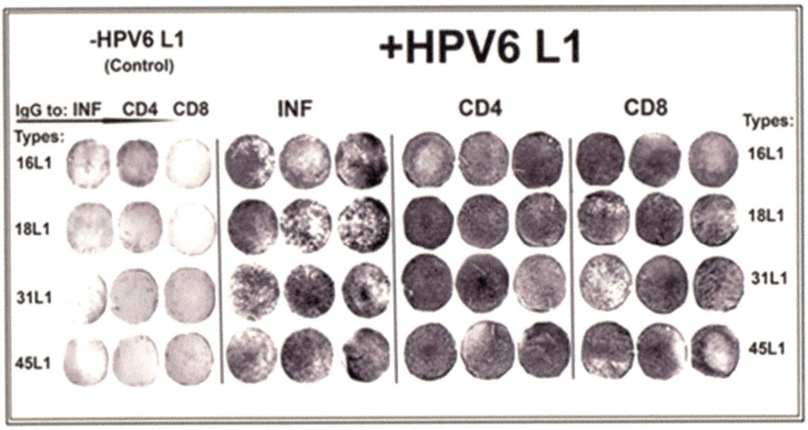

Figure 5.
The induction of the synthesis of interferon (INF), CD4 and CD8 T lymphocytes in peripheral mononuclear blood cells from mice orally vaccinated with vaccines of antigenic HPV16, 18, 31 and 45 L1 by another antigenic protein of phylogenetically unrelated type of papillomavirus HPV6 L1. Control - the inoculation of T lymphocytes from blood of corresponding variants of vaccinated mice was without HPV6 L1.

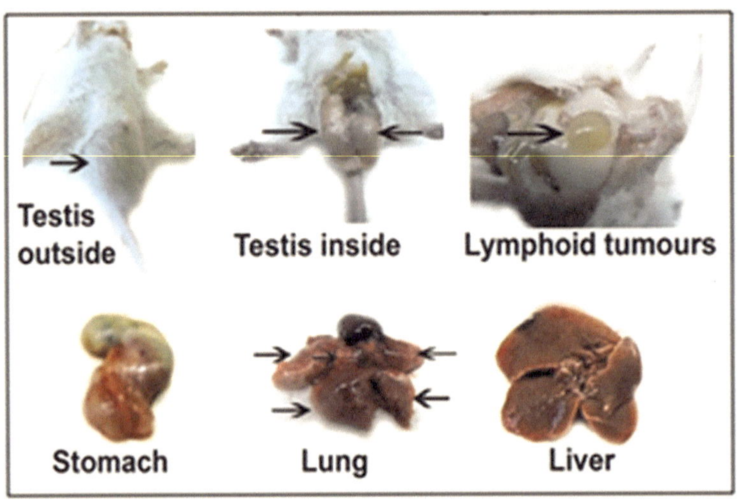

Figure 6.
Tumour formation in mice bodies after 1 month of the injection of cancer HeLa cells. Arrows indicate tumours.

The effect of the injection of HeLa cells on the morphology of lungs of mice (both male and female) and the regression of the morphology changing after oral vaccination with vaccine material of tomato fruit with "early" protein HPV16 E2 could be seen in **Figure 10**. Control variant (+HeLa-E2) of mice lungs without treatment – mice lungs after 2 months after the injection with HeLa cells and vaccination with HPV16 E2. Variant (+HeLa+E2) - mice lungs after 2 months after the injection with HeLa cells and then after 2 months of double vaccination with HPV16 E2 with the interval of 1 month. Lungs of mice only vaccinated with HPV16 E2 were without any changes (not shown in **Figure 10**). Lungs were presented together with hearts because of easier manipulation with them by holding hearts with tweezers.

DOI: http://dx.doi.org/10.5772/intechopen.1001912

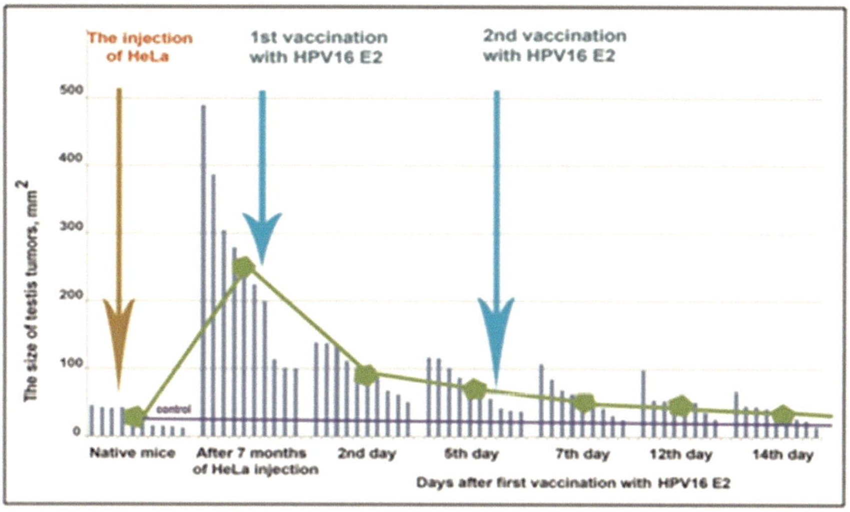

Figure 7.
The regression of testis tumours in male mice after the vaccination with HPV16 E2. N = 10 mice.

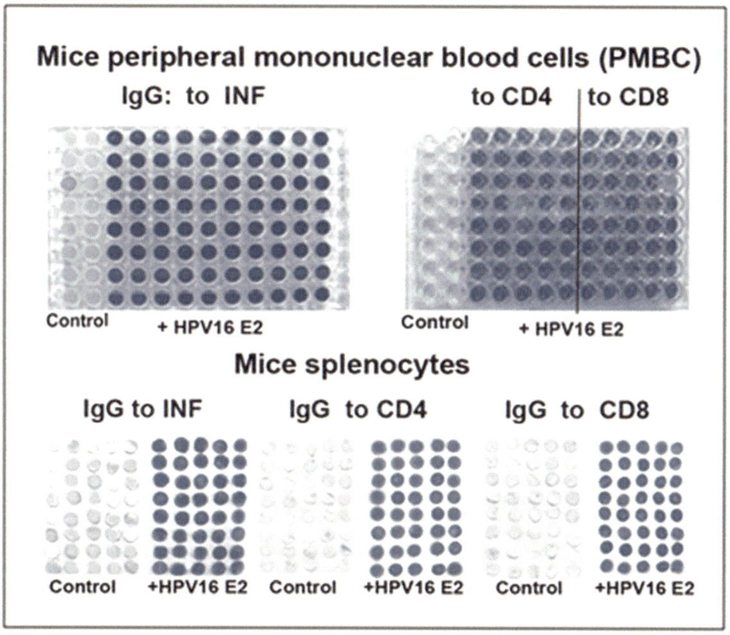

Figure 8.
The Elispot (left and bottom) and ELISA (upper right) analyses the increase of the synthesis of interferon (INF) and enlarging of generations of CD4/CD8 T lymphocytes both in PMBC and splenocytes. Control - without HPV16 E2.

When it was found that the one-time incubation of isolated mice lungs with HeLa cells and HPV16 E2 cancelled the formation of the tumours in isolated mice lungs and oral vaccination with HPV16 E2 abolished the tumour formation and resulted in tumour regression, it was decided to analyse the direct action of HPV16 E2, E6, E7, LAAO and DAAO on growing cancer HeLa cells. The action was estimated by using the staining with trypan blue dye-coloured dead cells because of the destruction of cell membranes.

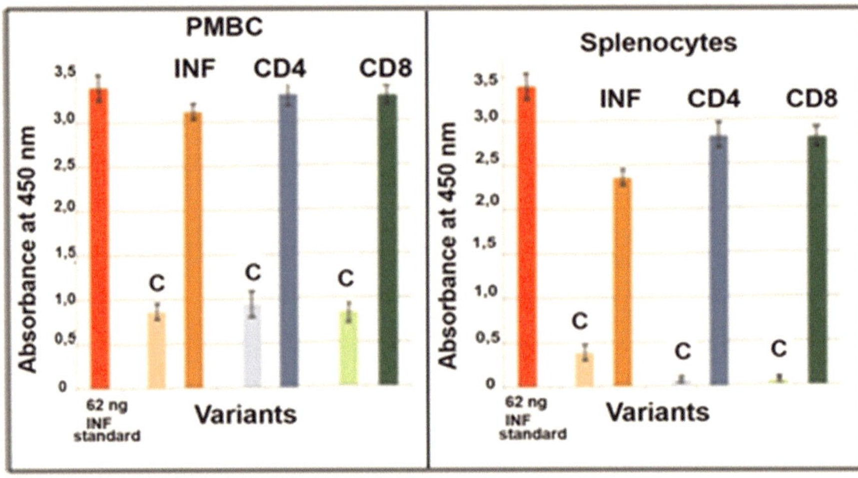

Figure 9.
ELISA analysis of the contents of INF, CD4/CD8 T lymphocytes after in PMBC and splenocytes of mice orally vaccinated with tomato vaccine material with HPV16 E2. C-control [15].

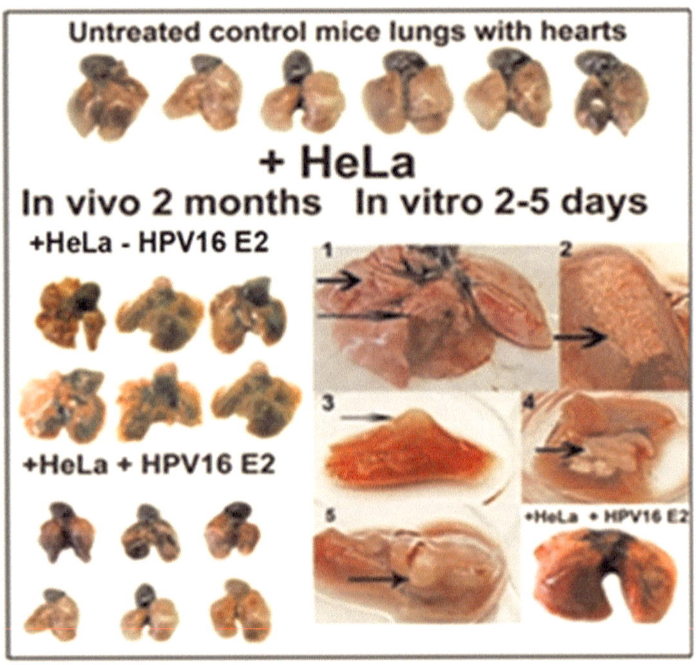

Figure 10.
The sensitivity of mice lungs to the inoculation with HeLa cells. №№ 1–5 - tumours of different types observed on the surface of isolated mice lungs after 2–5 days of inoculation with HeLa cells. The oral vaccination with HPV16 E2 of mice previously incubated with HeLa cells abolished the tumour formation in isolated mice lung (to the right bottom), variant +HeLa+HPV16 E2.

As can be seen from **Figure 11**, antigenic proteins HPV16 E6 and HPV16 E7 did not influence HeLa cells (№ 2 and № 3), but HPV16 E2, LAAO and DAAO killed HeLa cells because the trypan blue dye showed dark blue colour and destroyed cell structures (cell debris) appeared.

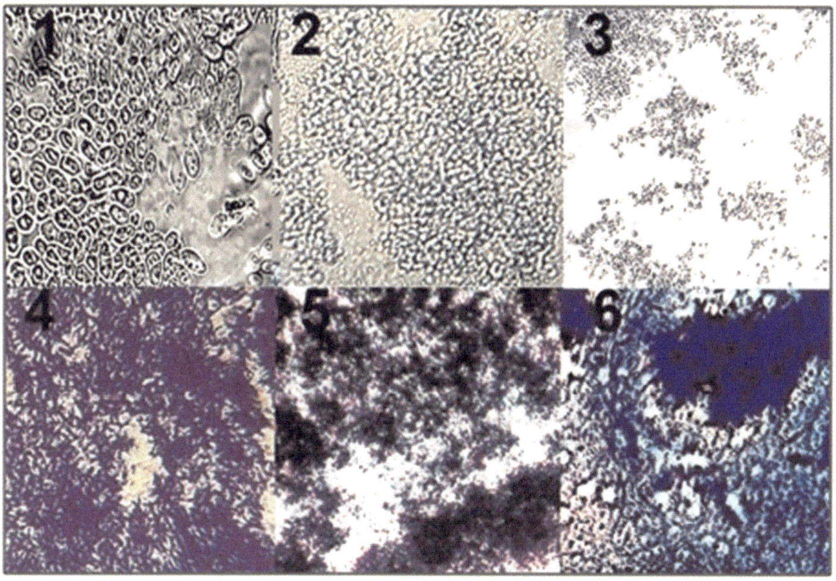

Figure 11.
The effect of the "early" proteins HPV16 E2, E6, E7, LAAO and DAAO on cancer HeLa cells. 1 - cells of fresh-grown suspension of HeLa cells, 2 - HeLa cells in the presence of HPV16 E6 and trypan blue (TB), 3 - the absence of staining of HeLa cells with TB in the presence of HPV16 E7, 4 - the full destruction of HeLa cells and staining with TB after the addition of the HPV16 E2, 5 - the destruction of HeLa cells and of staining with TB in the presence of LAAO, 6 - the destruction of HeLa cells and staining with TB in the presence of DAAO.

Tumour overgrowths cones and waves of cell proliferation with dark-coloured hyperchromic nuclei that could be seen in **Figure 12** were analogs of small-round-cell lung sarcoma with hyperchromic stained nuclei.

In **Figure 13**, it could be seen patterns of normal lung tissues: flattened cells of peripheral lung parenchima with faintly coloured nuclei, patterns of smooth muscle elongated cells and their transverse sections with pale coloured nuclei of myocytes, patterns of bronchioles elements, loose connective tissue cells with rare hyperchromic nuclei. There were no huge proliferative areas of dividing cells with hyperchromic stained nuclei into slices made of normal lung tissues without HeLa. In order to study immunogenic and oncolytic activities of HPV16 E2, peripheral mononuclear blood cells (PMBC) and splenocytes orally vaccinated with the HPV16 E2 tomato vaccine were isolated according to methods [17, 18].

As it was seen from **Figures 14** and **15**, (**Table A2**) the oral vaccination mice with vaccine material containing antigenic protein HPV16 E2 highly increased the synthesis of γ-interferon, accelerated the generation of CD4/CD8 T lymphocytes and activated apoptotic enzymes: granzyme B, perforin and granulysin.

In attempts to decipher the oncolytic effect of HPV16 E2, the Elispot analysis with antibodies to protein inhibitors of check-point control of carcinogenesis was undertaken with antibodies to the receptor on T lymphocytes PD-1 and to cancer receptor PD-L1 (**Figure 16**) (**Tables A3** and **A4**).

To obtain these results, fresh isolated mice lungs (12 mice at the age of 6 months and masses of 35–40 g) were placed in Corning flasks with DMEM nutritive medium in which cancer HeLa cells were grown. At this time, the solution of antibodies to PD-1 and PD-L1 (each 10 μl) was put in the flasks. Flasks were left for 2 days until tumour overgrows became visible on the surface of the lungs.

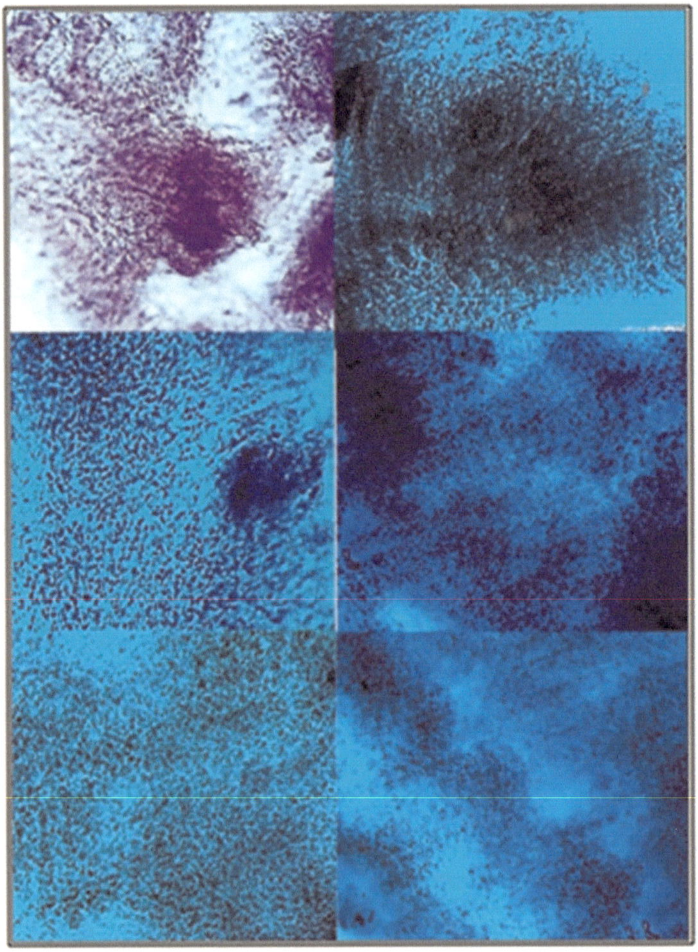

Figure 12.
Patterns of microtome slices of mice lungs after 5 days of inoculation with cancer HeLa cells (variant +HeLa-E2) without vaccination. Slices were stained with haematoxylin by Carazzi.

Then lungs were minced with a syringe needle in 1 ml of DMEM, and homogenates were placed in a centrifuge tube and floated at 700 g for 7 minutes at 4°C as described in [16–18]. Aliquots of 20 μl were added to wells of Corning microplate (25 wells) on nitrocellulose disks (12 mm in diameter) with 300 μl of DMEM. 100 μg of the water solution (100 μl) of HPV16 E2 was placed, and the incubation was continued for 5 days. After that, the procedure was as follows [17, 18]. It was found that when the cancer checkpoint was inhibited with antibody to PD-L1, HPV16 E2 highly activated the formation of T cell receptors (TCR) and increased the activity of apoptotic enzymes: granzyme B, perforine and granulysin.

As a matter of fact, as a whole, the immune system of mice lungs appeared to be less active up to 100 times (at least) than it was in the spleen or in PMBC. Gentle mice lung cells might be unable to resist the invasion of HeLa cells and not survive. Nevertheless, the addition of HPV16 E2 effectively increased the synthesis of interferon (INF), T cell receptors (TCR) and accelerated the generation of CD/CD8 T lymphocytes, even in lung T lymphocytes damaged with HeLa cells.

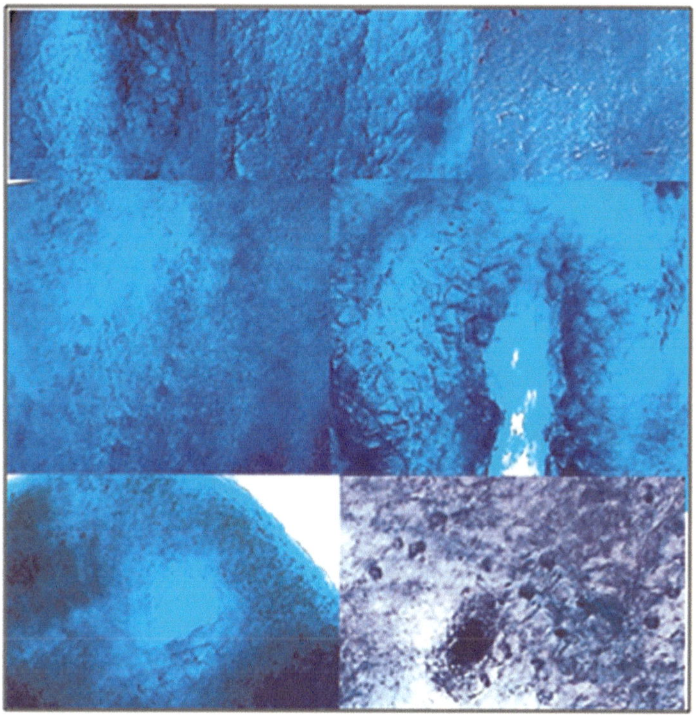

Figure 13.
Patterns of microtome slices of mice lungs after 5 days of the inoculation with cancer HeLa cells in the presence of vaccine material of tomato fruit transgenic with HPV16 E2 (variant +HeLa+E2). Slices were stained with haematoxylin by Carazzi.

LAAO and DAAO appeared to have immunogenic activities (**Figure 17**) (**Tables A5** and **A6**) in blood and spleen isolated from mice.

To appreciate the immunogenic and oncolytic effectivities of L-amino acid and D-amino acid oxidases (LAAO and DAAO), the experimental design was employed as follows: fresh isolated mice lungs (at the age of 6 months with masses 35–40 g) was placed in Corning flasks with the suspension of growing cancer HeLa cells per 1 day. Tumours of overgrowths appeared on the surface of the lungs the next day after placing of lungs into flasks (**Figure 18**). To flasks, 10 mg of LAAO or DAAO in DMEM solution were added separately. On the next day after oxidase addition, the tumours became smaller and later disappeared on 5th–6th days of inoculation, revealing a smooth surface. These lungs were used in Elispot analysis to evaluate the immunogenic activities of LAAO and DAAO (**Figure 19**).

In order to understand what happened with a large area of lungs with tumour cells having hyperchromic nuclei, the microtome slices were prepared (**Figure 20**).

There were not found widespread areas of round cancer cells having hyperchromic nuclei in microtomic slices prepared from lungs at first inoculated with HeLa and after being treated with LAAO. There were presented cells, and tissues resembled patterns of smooth muscle elongated cells with pale coloured nuclei of myocytes, flattened cells of peripheral lung parenchyma with faintly coloured nuclei, and loose connective tissue cells with rare hyperchromic nuclei. Alveolocytes (A) and bronchioles (bronchi) clearly could be seen (**Figure 20**).

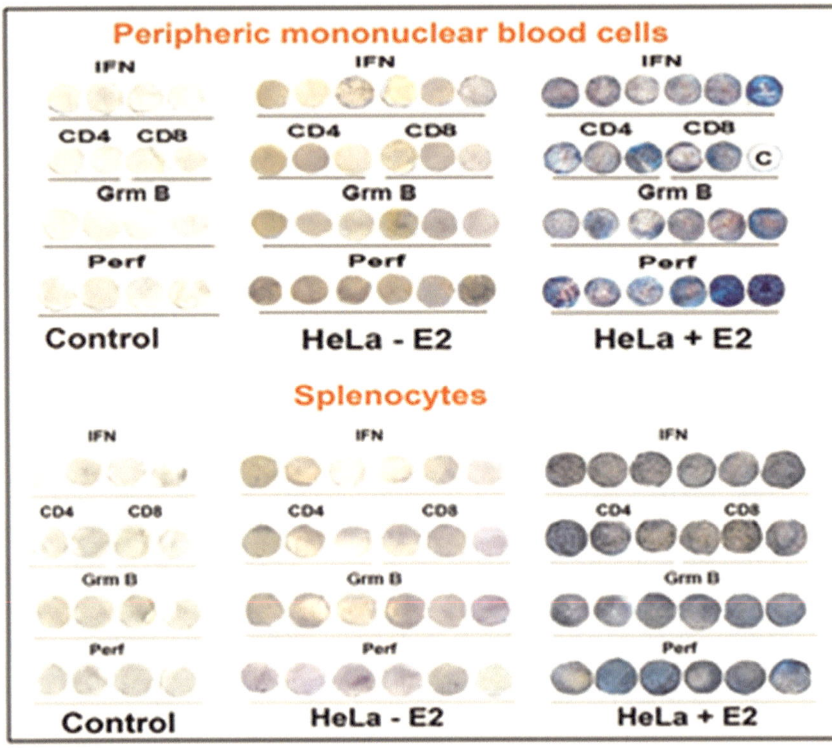

Figure 14.
Elispot analysis of the activation of the synthesis of interferon (INF), CD4 and CD8 T lymphocytes, apoptotic enzymes: Granzyme B (GrmB) and perforin (perf) in peripheral mononuclear blood cells and in splenocytes, preliminary injected with cancer HeLa cells and then vaccinated with vaccine material of tomato fruit with transgenic HPV16 E2. Letter "C" means control [17, 18]. Control - without any treatment.

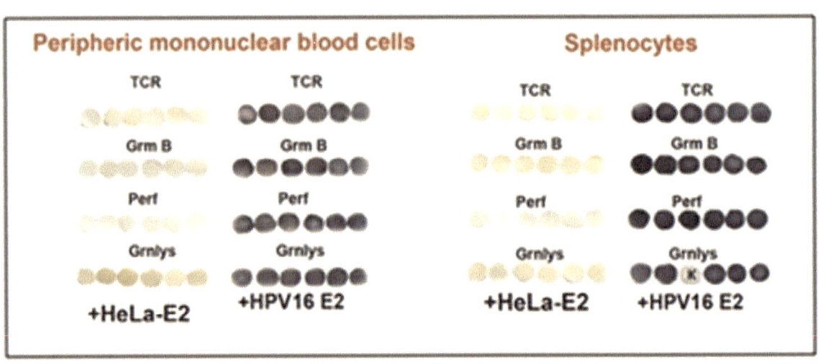

Figure 15.
Elispot analysis of the activation of the synthesis of T cell receptors (TCR) and apoptotic enzymes: Granzyme B (GrmB), perforin (perf) and granulysin (Grnlys) in peripheral mononuclearblood cells and in splenocytes of mice injected with cancer HeLa cells and then vaccinated with vaccine material of tomato fruit transgenic with HPV16 E2. Control (+HeLa-E2) - mice injected with cancer HeLa cells without vaccination. Letter "K" in the lower row to the right means empty membrane disk without adding of splenocytes.

From the results presented in **Figures 18–20**, (**Table A7**) it might be concluded that L-amino acid oxidase (LAAO) and D-amino acid oxidase (DAAO) both were active as activators (effectors) of the immune response in peripheral mononuclear blood cells and in splenocytes. But their actions were more pronounced on the mice lung T lymphocytes

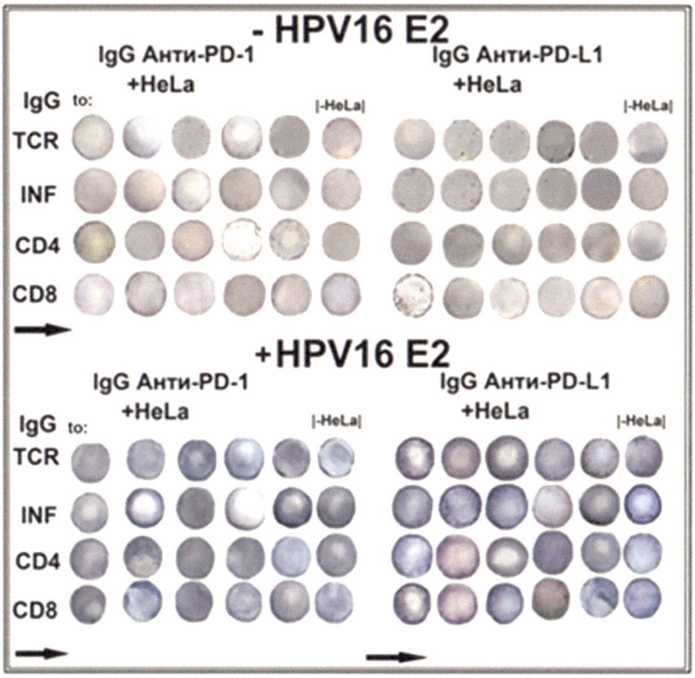

Figure 16.
Elispot amalyses of the activation of immune response in colonies of T lymphocytes isolated from mice lungs after the inoculation in the suspension of HeLa cells in the presence of antibodies to check-points PD-1 and PD-L1 evoked by vaccine material of tomato fruit transgenic with HPV16 E2. (see details in the text).

treated with cancer HeLa cells. This is the first evidence of the activity of LAAO and DAAO on the immune system and especially on the immune system of mice lungs after the invasion of cancer HeLa cells. This observation is in good correlation with the results of **Table 1** in that it was shown the predicted antigenic determinants for T cells (HLA-B13 decamers) determined with the database SYFPEITHI. Both LAAO and DAAO have potent epitopes but without any similarity to other antigenic proteins used in this study.

4. Discussion

As a matter of fact, lungs are chronically exposed to an array of cellular and airborne stressors, including aerosols, infectious agents, allergens, pollutants, pneumotoxic chemicals, medications and other biomedical injuries. To overcome these biological and environmental stresses, the lungs must make lower the immune response as a whole [19]. Pulmonary lipoproteins have been shown to modulate the inflammatory response to microbial components. These surfactants were able to inhibit macrophage proinflammatory cytokine response and reduced inflammatory mediator production by blocking the toll-like receptor 2 (TLR2) pathways, thus repressing lung inflammation caused by internal stresses [20]. For example, pulmonary surfactants are complex and highly surface-active materials that are found in the fluid lining of the alveolar surface and play an important role in stabilising breathing, pulmonary homeostasis and mucosal immunity [20]. Human surfactant protein D (SP-D) facilitates SARS-Cov-2 pseudotype binding, and entry with pattern recognition receptors having the crucial immune

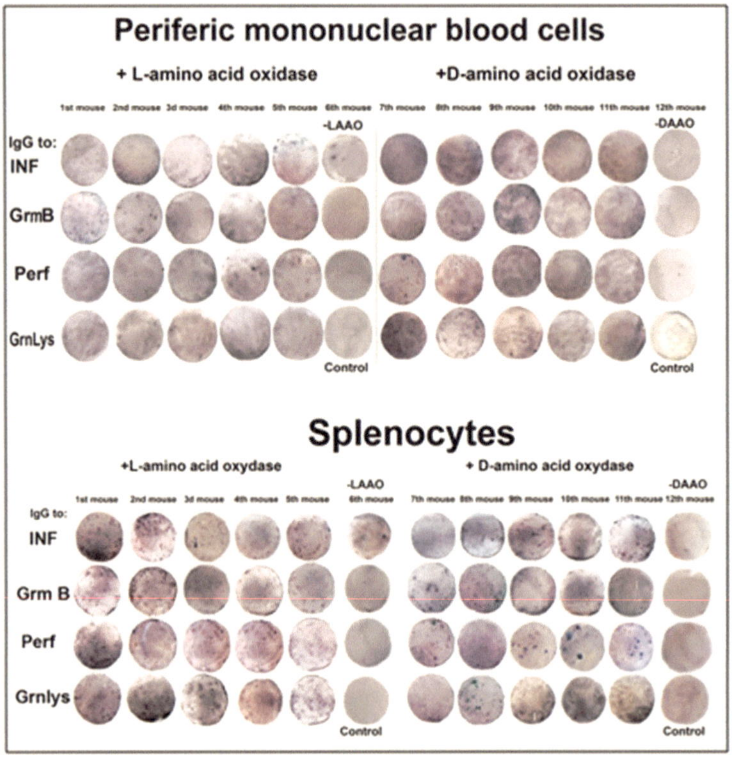

Figure 17.
Elispot analysis of immunogenic activity of LAAO and DAAO in PMBC and splenocytes of untreated mice.

function in detecting, and clearing pulmonary pathogens and downregulates spike protein-induced inflammation [21]. Recombinant fragments of human SP-D having comparable immunological activities to native SP-D binds to gp120 and inhibit HIV-1 infectivity and replication in monocytic cells, Jurkat T cells and peripheral mononuclear blood cells inhibiting HIV-1 triggered cytokine storm. The immune surveillance role of SP-D in terms of its ability to recognise viruses and modulate unwanted inflammatory responses was considered broadly in relation to HIV-1 infection and SARS-Cov-2 diseases [21]. But there are no studies aimed at investigating the multiple HPV abnormalities at all in the lungs in the light of pulmonary pattern recognition receptors. As well as, nobody paid attention to the events predetermining carcinogenesis of the lungs in the case of HPV or HeLa cancer cells infectivities.

It was shown the result of inoculation of male mice with HeLa cells evidencing at least 10 times increase in the area of the testis in **Figures 6** and 7 during a month. This might occur due to cell surface receptor transmembrane heparan sulphate proteoglycan syndecan-1, which is critically involved in the differentiation and propagation of various tumours [22]. The syndecan-1 protein is a receptor situated in the equatorial region of the sperm head that specifically binds to the papillomavirus coat protein L of the "late" expression and therefore has a poor influence on male fertility [23]. Possibly, this explains the active proliferation of HeLa cells and tumour overgrowths in the testis area. The oral vaccination with HPV16 E2 protein of infected male mice has a clearly detectable antiproliferative effect, causing a pronounced regression of testicular tumours in male mice.

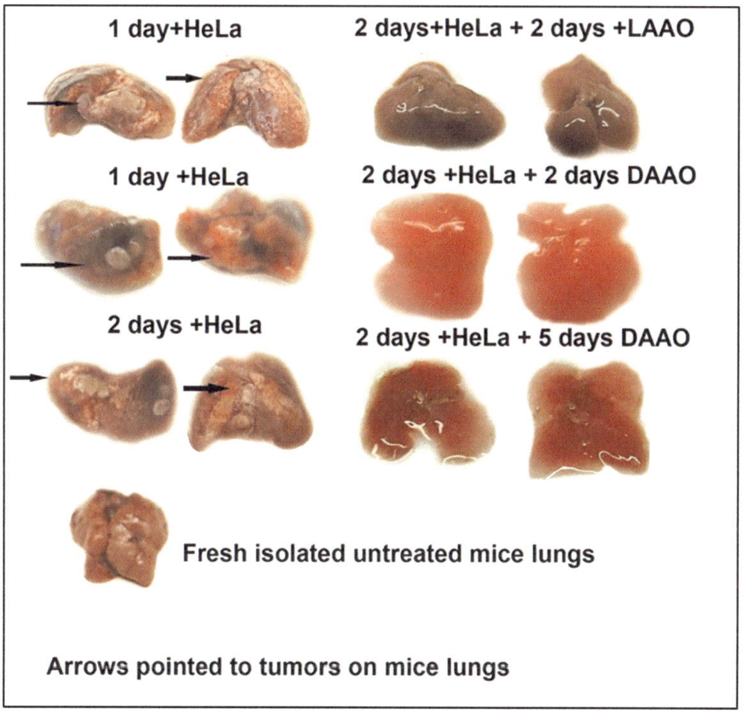

Figure 18.
The effect of LAAO and DAAO on tumours of mice lungs evoked by cancer HeLa cells.

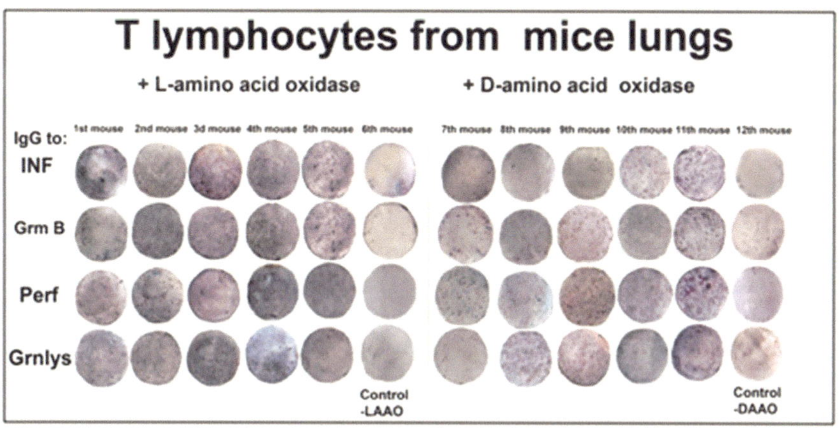

Figure 19.
Elispot analysis of LAAO and DAAO immunogenic activity in T lymphocytes isolated from mice lungs inoculated with cancer HeLa cells.

The "early" expression HPV16 E2 protein has attracted the attention of other researchers [24]. By studying the structure and activity of the E2 protein, it was found that the E2 protein is a powerful repressor of the promoter from which the viral oncogenes HPV16 E6 and HPV16 E7 are transcribed. The E2 protein included two domains: a transactivation N-domain and a DNA-binding C domain. The N-terminal domain of the E2 protein is fused to a hinge, and the E8 gene product forms a complex called the E2C domain. The whole structure of E2C of joined E8^E2 proteins interacts

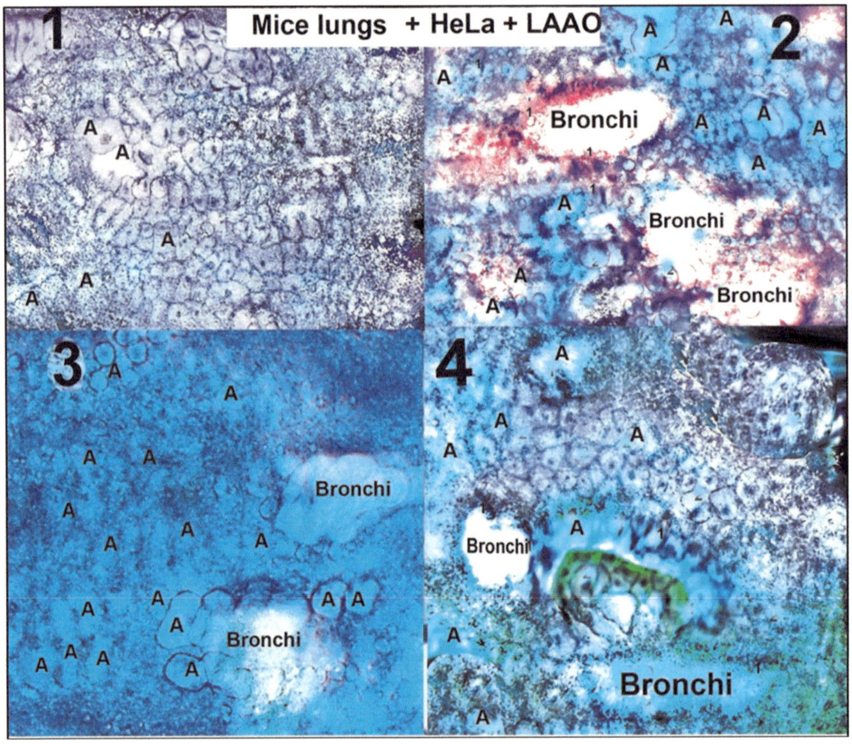

Figure 20.
*Microtomic slices prepared from lungs treated at first with cancer HeLa cells and after inoculated with LAAO (from **Figure 19**, upper right). 1–4 - microtomic slices, A-alveolocytes, bronchi - bronchioles.*

with a common nuclear repressor complex in host cells. The dysregulation of the repressor complex causes different types of carcinogenesis [24].

During rapid infection of murine lungs, it might exist the receptor or complexes of proteins like well-known pattern recognition pathogen receptors on the surface area of alveolocytes. Toll-like receptors play an important role in the natural defences against virus infection. However, they may promote inflammation events related to cancer development. The interaction between TLR4/TLR9 gene polymorphisms and HPV16/18 infection influencing cervical lesion risk was shown in [25].

Different protease families are found on the plasma membrane in the secretory pathways of cells and widely expressed in the nasopharinx, respiratory tracts and so on, where they are involved in the tropism and pathogenesis of coronaviruses, influenza viruses and other respiratory viruses, hopefully as well as human papillomaviruses. Moreover, proteases play an important role in viral maturation by processing many polyproteins that are translated from the viral RNA [26], with the evidence obtained from various experiments supporting the notion that proteases can be a viable antiviral target for COVID-19. So proteases are promising drug targets for antiviral treatment (COVID-19 et cetera). Still, the drug development and therapeutics toward them could be a very complicated process taking into account the efficacy and toxicity of proteases modulating at the enzymatic, cellular, organ and as well as system levels [26]. The developing effective yet low-toxicity treatment and mild preventive therapies might be considered the use of L-amino acid oxidase or D-amino acid oxidase that have antibacterial, antiviral, anticancer and antiproliferative properties [27] and are showing highly immunogenic and oncolytic behaviour according to our data obtained with the treatment of murine lungs tumours with LAAO and DAAO. These results are worthy of attention and continuation of the investigation.

According to the above considered, the native loss of immune defence might be the reason for the missed immunity resulting to the rapid tumour formation at the next day of the placing of murine lungs in suspension of HeLa cells in our experiments.

5. Conclusion

Murine peripheral mononuclear blood cells, splenocytes and lungs were considered to be excellent experimental models to discover the immune response of cell immunity and the induction of immune T lymphocytes to different antigenic and therapeutic proteins. Furthermore, having adult healthy mice in the laboratory, one can appreciate the immune response of protein of interest during a week using the standard Elispot technique.

As it was found that murine lungs are very gentle of mice internal organs with a high inclination to tumour formation without strong defence by humeral or cells systems and are able very fast to form tumours overgrowths, murine lungs appeared to be the appropriate object for rapid screening of immune antigenic and oncolytic proteins, as well as substances with high oncogenic potentiality. Therefore, the whole procedure continued for 5–7 days in order to investigate the activity of proteins and therapeutics of interest.

Appendix: supplement

Tables A1–A7

HPV type	Control			Experience		
	IFN*	CD4*	CD8*	IFN*	CD4*	CD8*
16	128	108	72	1980, 1800, 1220	1120, 1182, 1230	1980, 2016, 1186
18	98	78	76	1240, 1450, 1560	1840, 1684, 1208	1360, 2000, 1820
31	240	132	208	1160, 1950, 1420	1760, 1620, 1800	1185, 1560, 1670
45	204	15	36	1680, 1720, 1850	1860, 1840, 1380	1960, 1820, 1920

**Antibodies to INF, CD4 and CD8 T lymphocytes were used in analyses.*

Table A1.
The inductison of the synthesis of interferon (INF), CD4 and CD8 T lymphocytes in peripheral mononuclear blood cells from mice vaccinated with vaccines of antigenic HPV16, 18, 31 and 45 L1 by another antigenic protein of phylogenetically unrelated type of papillomavirus HPV6 L1.

Variant	γ-Interferon	CD4	CD8	Granzyme B	Perforin
Peripheral mononuclear blood cells (PMBC)					
Control	5, 20, 17, 14	8, 9, 0	5, 4, 0	6, 7, 10, 7	0, 2, 5, 14
+HeLa-E2	6, 10, 22, 3, 0, 51	7, 8, 4	12, 4, 14	8, 2, 8,17, 9, 5	41,6,4,7,5,8
+HeLa+E2	420, 840, 584, 512, 576,460	615, 1232, 615	646, 1104	688, 924, 672, 840, 749, 720	760, 666, 1007, 552, 491, 354

Variant	γ-Interferon	CD4	CD8	Granzyme B	Perforin
Splenocytes					
Control	0, 6, 12, 0	1, 5	7, 0	6, 0, 0, 0	0,6,6, 0
+HeLa-E2	9, 7, 0,14,43, 53	57, 25,16	9, 21, 7	14,44, 36, 28, 0,5	30, 15, 10 11, 14,11
+HeLa+E2	448, 568, 664, 280, 680, 572	600,642, 595	511, 504, 336	570, 384, 540, 590, 564, 264	435, 485, 528, 618, 612, 552

Table A2.
Therapeutic action of HPV16 E2 on the content of γ-interferon, amount of CD4 and CD8 T lymphocytes, granzyme B and perforin in blood and spleen of mice, preliminary intramuscular injected with HeLa cells (amount of cells was presented in account per membrane nitrocellulose filter). Figures corresponded to individual mice (here and further 1 figure =1 mice).

Variant	TCR	Granzyme B	Perforin	Granulysin
Peripheral mononuclear blood cells (PMBC)				
+HeLa -E2	31, 20, 14, 27, 16, 23	33, 41, 15, 25,37, 39	44, 30, 9, 23, 25, 27	15, 19, 13, 20, 22, 25
+HeLa +E2	1224, 2512, 4688, 1892, 2800, 2312	1084, 1691, 4466, 4912, 5104, 6945	3532, 4280, 5120, 5216, 3248, 4096	5364, 4688, 4480, 4234, 5016, 4896
Splenocytes				
+HeLa - E2	32, 40, 24, 10, 26, 9	40, 74, 59, 39, 45, 53	18, 15, 32, 20, 25, 26	18, 15, 13, 12, 19, 13
+HeLa + E2	824, 1165, 864, 964, 896, 1176	1008, 1104, 634, 952, 1004, 1126	1480, 1304, 1392, 1384, 1064, 1392	1648, 1220, 992, 1360, 1088

Table A3.
The therapeutic action of HPV16 E2 on the content of T cell receptor (TCR), granzyme B, perforine and granulysine in peripheric mononuclear blood cells and splenocytes of mice, preliminary intramuscular injected with HeLa cells.

Variant of IgG to:	Anti PD-1 IgG - E2		Anti PD-L1 IgG - E2	
	+HeLa	-HeLa	+HeLa	-HeLa
The number of stained immunopositive colonies of T lymphocytes (immune "spots")				
TCR	19, 20, 30, 40, 5	31	18, 27, 30, 38, 5	23
INF	11, 20, 25, 3, 2	29	23, 46, 35, 25, 17	25
CD4	26, 16, 4, 20, 24	22	3, 16, 16, 12, 16	34
CD8	21, 14, 7, 5, 15	15	55, 31, 29, 9, 19	20
Anti D-1 IgG + HPV16 E2		Anti PD-L1 IgG + HPV16 E2		
TCR	156, 174, 104, 105, 133	63	400, 210, 223, 304, 187	168
INF	185, 156, 147, 127, 63	31	169, 484, 195, 198, 238	260
CD4	213, 228, 119, 106, 97	56	178, 145, 143, 274, 156	428
CD8	169, 103, 170, 220, 127	96	210, 145, 195, 105,159	456

Table A4.
The content of colour immunopositive colonies of T lymphocytes isolated from mice lungs inoculated with the suspension of HeLa cells in the presence of antibodies to inhibitors of checkpoints PD-1 and PD-L1, activated by adding the effector HPV16 E2 from tomato fruit.

IgG to:	+L-amino acid oxidase	Control* -LAAO	+D-amino acid oxidase	Control* -DAAO
INF	84, 128, 96, 116, 88	10	168, 118, 108, 117, 140	37
GrmB	92, 128, 100, 138, 172	16	96, 108, 132, 128, 96	35
Perf	92, 112, 84, 92, 76	22	140, 125, 124, 92, 76	31
Grnlys	88, 104, 80, 104, 64	37	116, 292, 100, 104, 104	30

**- Mice PMBC without any treatment used as control ones.*

Table A5.
The activation of the synthesis of interferon (INF), granzyme B (Grm B), perforin (perf) and granulysin (Grnlys) in T lymphocytes isolated from mice periferic mononuclear blood cells PMBC) after the addition of L-amino acid oxidase (LAAO) or of D-amino acid oxidase (DAAO).

IgG to:	+ L-amino acid oxidase	Control* -LAAO	+ D-amino acid oxidase	Control* -DAAO
INF	163, 174, 224, 105, 165	14	201, 179, 85, 152, 268	42
Grm B	141, 243, 144, 144, 149	12	186, 190, 142, 155, 336	58
Perf	119, 132, 126, 126, 221	67	191, 164, 103, 120, 184	59
Grnlys	231, 134, 102, 102, 93	15	73, 160, 158, 176, 224	56

**- Isolated splenocytes from mice spleen without any treatment used as control ones.*

Table A6.
The activation of the synthesis of interferon (INF), granzyme B (Grm B), perforin (perf) and granulysin (Grnlys) in T lymphocytes (splenocytes) isolated from mice spleen after the addition of L-amino acid oxidase (LAAO) or of D-amino acid oxidase (DAAO).

IgG to:	+L-amino acid oxidase	Control -LAAO	+D-amino acid oxidase	Control -DAAO
INF	376, 504, 364, 372, 364	29	456, 146, 160, 380, 370	53
GrmB	392, 492, 444, 368, 268	37	160, 280, 380, 372, 332	58
Perf	670, 336, 268, 332, 332	47	288, 352, 560, 436, 516	61
Grnlys	392, 364, 336, 348, 348	38	216, 336, 445, 103, 236	45

Table A7.
The content of immunospots in T lymphocytes isolated from mice lungs inoculated with cancer HeLa after treating with L-amino acid oxidase (LAAO) or with D-amino acid oxidase (DAAO).

Author details

Natalya Rekoslavskaya*, Rurik Salyaev and Alexey Stolbikov
Siberian Institute of Plant Physiology and Biochemistry of the Siberian Branch of Russian Academy of Sciences, Irkutsk, Russian Federation

*Address all correspondence to: rekoslavskaya@sifibr.irk.ru

References

[1] Kim R, Emi M, Tanabe K. Cancer immunoediting from immune surveillance to immune escape. Immunology. 2007;**121**:1-14. DOI: 10.1111/j.1365-2567.2007.02587.x

[2] Siegel RL, Hiller D, Wagle NS, Jemal A. Cancer statistics, 2023. CA: A Cancer Journal for Clinicians. 2023;**73**: 17-48. DOI: 10.3322/caac.21763

[3] Poizot-Martin J, Henry M, Benhaim S, Obry-Roget V, Figarella D, Tamalet C. High level of HPV16 and 18 DNA level in anal swabs from male and female HIV-1 infected patients. Journal of Clinical Virology. 2009;**44**:314-317. DOI: 10.1016/jcv.2009.02.003

[4] Smirnov VS, Kudryavtseva TA. Treatment of human papillomaviruses infection in HIV-infected patients. Russian Journal of Infection and Immunity. 2021;**11**:79-84. DOI: 10.15789/2220-7619-TOH-1233

[5] Kumar BV, Connors T, Farber DL. Human T cell development, localization, and function throughout life. Immunity. 2018;**48**:202-213. DOI: 10.1016/j.immuni.2018.01.007

[6] Strebel PM, Papania MJ, Gastanaduy PA, Goodson JL. Plotkin's vaccines. Seventh ed. Amsterdam: Elsevier; 2018. pp. 579-618. e.21. DOI: 10.1016/B978-0-35761-6.00037-7

[7] Lythe G, Callard RE, Hoare RL, Molina-Paris C. How many TCR clonotypes does a body maintain? Journal of Theoretical Biology. 2016; **389**:214-224. DOI: 10.1016/j.jtbi.2015.10.016

[8] Tough DF, Sprent J. Lifespan of naive and memory T cells. Stem Cells. 1995;**13**: 242-249. DOI: 10.1002/stem.5530130305

[9] Macallan DC, Borghans JAM, Asquith B. Human T cell memory: A dynamic view. Vaccine. 2017;**5**:1-12. DOI: 10.3390/vaccines5010005

[10] Garbuglia AR, Lapa D, Sias D, Capabiachi MR, Del Porto P. The use of both therapeutic and prophylactic vaccines in the therapy of papillomavirus disease. Frontiers in immunology. 2020; **1**. Article 18:1-14. DOI: 10.3389/fimmu.2020.00188

[11] Beltran ORC, Ledezma RR. MVA E2 therapeutic vaccine for marked reduction in likelyhood of recurrent respiratory papillomatosis. Head & Neck. 2019;**41**:657-665. DOI: 10.1002/hed.244777

[12] Salyaev R, Rekoslavskaya N, Stolbikov A. The new plant expression system for the creation of vaccines against papillomaviruses. Doklady. Biochemistry and Biophysics. 2019;**484**: 52-54. DOI: 10.1134/S1607672919010150

[13] Salyaev R, Rekoslavskaya N, Stolbikov A. Synthesis of proteins encoded by the early genes E2, E6 and E7 of papillomavirus of type 16 in the plant expression system. Doklady. Biochemistry and Biophysics. 2018;**482**: 271-274. DOI: 10.1134/S160767291 8050113

[14] Salyaev R, Rekoslavskaya N. The use of the antigenic protein HPV6 L1 to induce the synthesis of interferon, CD4 and CD8 T lymphocytes, and granzyme B in blood and splenocytes of mice in order to develop a broad vaccine against dangerous papillomatoses. Doklady. Biochemistry and Biophysics. 2021;**500**:331-335. DOI: 10.1134/S160767292105015X

[15] Salyaev R, Rekoslavskaya N, Stolbikov A. The antiproliferative effect

of the "early" protein E2 of papillomavirus HPV16 on testis tumors of mice induced by the injection of HeLa cells. Doklady. Biochemistry and Biophysics. 2019;**488**:296-299. DOI: 10.1134/S16076729190028

[16] Salyaev R, Rekoslavskaya N, Stolbikov A. The induction of the synthesis of interferon, CD4 and CD8 T lymphocytes in blood and spleen of mice after oral vaccination with the "early" protein HPV16 E2. Doklady. Biochemistry and Biophysics. 2019;**488**: 316-319. DOI: 10.1134/S16076729 19050077

[17] Salyaev R, Rekoslavskaya N. The effect of "early" proteins E2, E6 and E7 of papillmavirus of high-risk cancerogenous type HPV16 on HeLa cells inducing tumour growth in mice lungs. Acta Biomedica Scientifica. 2022; 7:260-276. DOI: 10.29413/ABS.2022-7.3.26

[18] Salyaev R, Rekoslavskaya N, Stolbikov A. New data on the influence of the HPV16 E2 early protein obtained in plant expression nanosystems on tumor tissues of female mice induced by injection of HeLa cancer cells in hip muscle. Nanotechnologies in Russia. 2020;**15**:516-512. DOI: 10.1134/S1995078020040138

[19] Schneider JL, Rowe JH, Garcia-de-Alba C, Kim CF, Sharpe AH. The aging lung: Physiology, disease and immunity. Cell. 2021;**184**:1920-2019. DOI: 10.1016/j.cell.2021.03.005

[20] Ji J, Sun L, Luo Z, Zhang Y, Xianzheng W, Liao Y, et al. Potential therapeutic application of pulmonary surfactant lipids in the host defence against respiratory viral infections. Frontiers in Immunology. 2021;**12**: Article 730022:1-8. DOI: 10.3389/fimmu.2021.730022

[21] Beirag N, Kumar C, Madan T, Shamji MH, Bulla R, Mitchell D, et al. Human surfactant protein D facilitates SARS COV-2 pseudotype binding and entry in DC-sign expressing cells and downregulates spike protein induced inflammation. Frontiers in Immunology. 2022;**488**:13. Article 960733:1-19. DOI: 10.3389/fimmu.2022.960733

[22] Szatmari T, Otvos R, Hjerpe A, Dobra K. Syndecan-1 in cancer: Implication of cell signalling, differentiation and prognostication. Disease Marker (Hindawi Publishing Corporation). 2015;**488**:1-13. Article ID 796052. DOI: 10.1155/2015/796052

[23] Foresta C, Patassini C, Bertoldo A, Menegazzo M, Francavilla F, Barzon L, et al. Mechanism of human papillomavirus binding to human spermatozoa and fertilizing ability of infected spermatozoa. PLoS One. 2011;**6**: e15036. DOI: 10.1371/journal.pone.0015036

[24] Dreer M, Fertey J, van de Poel S, Straub E, Madung J, Macek B, et al. Interaction of NCOR/SMRT repressor complexes with papillomavirus E8^E2C proteins inhibits viral replication. PLOS Pathogens. 2016;**12**:e1005556. DOI: 10.1371/journal.ppat.1005556

[25] Zhang C, Yang Z, Luo P, Ye M, Gong P, Gong Q, et al. Association of TLR4 and TLR9 gene polymorphism with the risk and progression of cervical lesions in HPV-infected women. Biomarkers in Medicine. 2023;**17**: 133-142. DOI: 10.2217/bmm-2022-0702 Epub. 2023 Apr25

[26] Luan B, Huynh T, Cheng X, Wang H-R. Targeting proteases for treating COVID-19. Journal of Proteome Research. 2020;**19**:4316-4326. DOI: 10.1021/acs.jproteome.0c00430

[27] Lukasheva EV, Efremova AA, Treshalina EM, Arinbasarova AY, Medentzev AG, Berezov TT. L-amino acid oxidases: Properties and molecular mechanisms of action. Biochemistry (Moscow). Supplement Series B. Biomedical Chem. 2011;5:337-345. DOI: 10.1134/S199075081104007X

Section 3

Advances in Antigen Testing

Chapter 7

Antibody-Antigen Binding Events: The Effects of Antibody Orientation and Antigen Properties on the Immunoassay Sensitivity

Vanessa Susini, Chiara Sanguinetti, Silvia Ursino, Laura Caponi and Maria Franzini

Abstract

The sensitivity of an immunoassay depends on a complex combination of the physicochemical characteristics of antigens, antibodies, and reaction surfaces, which are the main elements on which the analytical principle of this technique is based. Among these characteristics is possible to include the type of surfaces, the affinity and avidity constants of antibodies, as well as antigen properties. This chapter focuses on the importance of the capturing surface in determining the analytical sensitivity of an immunoassay. It is an established knowledge that the sensitivity of immunoassays is affected by the orientation, the valence, and the spatial distribution of the capturing antibody. In addition, the size and the number of epitopes on the antigens (monovalent or multivalent) can influence the performances of these assays. In this chapter, the authors discuss how the combination of these factors reflects on the sensitivity of immunoassays.

Keywords: antibody, antigens, ELISAs, LFIAs, immunoassay, oriented-binding, affinity, avidity

1. Introduction

Enzyme immunoassays are based on the use of antibodies (Abs) to detect specific antigens (Ags). Among them, the enzyme-linked immunosorbent assay (ELISA) is the most frequently used. ELISA is a heterogeneous enzyme immunoassay technique, where one of the reaction components is nonspecifically adsorbed or covalently bound to the surface of a solid phase; the latter being usually provided by 96-well or 384-well polystyrene plates. The most common approach to using the ELISA technique is the "sandwich" type in which the antigen is bound by a so-called "capture antibody" immobilized on the solid surface. Then, an enzyme-labeled antibody (Ab*) is added to form an Ab-Ag-Ab* sandwich. The immunocomplexes are revealed

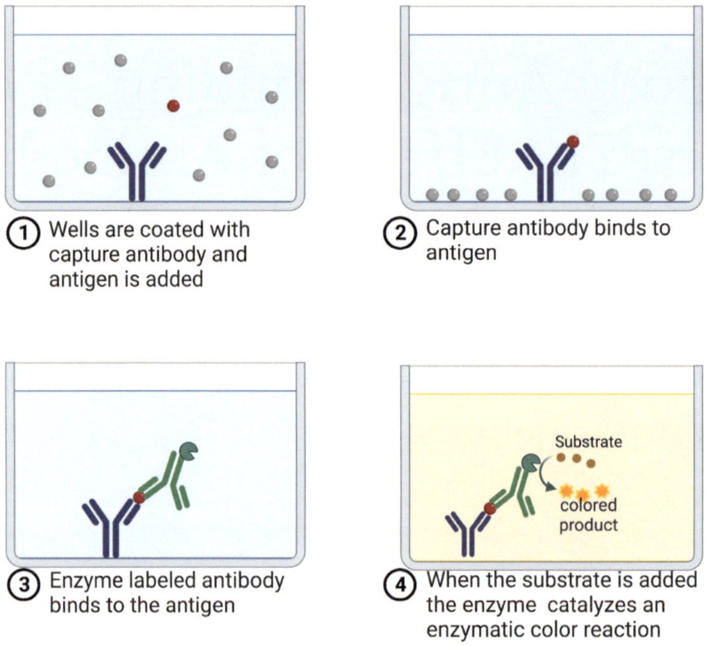

Figure 1.
Main phases of ELISA sandwich.

by adding the enzyme-substrate, which is converted to a detectable product whose amount is proportional to the quantity of Ag [1–3] (**Figure 1**).

ELISAs were first described in 1971 by Engvall and Perlmann as a rapid and sensitive method for detection and quantification of an antigen [4]. Today, this method is widely used in many different contexts, such as in clinical chemistry, environmental analysis, or quality control laboratories.

The lateral flow immunoassay (LFIA) or immunochromatographic strip is another widely used immunoassay format. Its success is mainly due to fast result (> 30 min), low development costs, and ease of production [5]. LFIAs contain all the required reagents within the strip itself that is usually supplied as a plastic cassette. The sample is loaded into a well that is in proximity to the conjugate pad containing the detection Abs that are conjugated with latex or gold microparticles. The Ags bind to the detection Abs and the so-formed immunocomplexes flow by capillary forces along a solid phase constituted by paper or nitrocellulose. The immunocomplexes are bound by the capturing Abs, which are coated on a specific region of the solid phase that is called "test line." The presence of the looked-for Ag is highlighted by the appearance of a colored line [3] (**Figure 2**). For a detailed description of LFIAs see Ref. [6].

LFIAs are used in medicine for the qualitative and quantitative detection of specific Ags, but they are also employed in veterinary medicine, food and environmental science, and even by police forces and regulatory authorities for the rapid detection of drugs [5].

The wide use of both ELISAs and LFIAs justifies the many ongoing studies aimed at improving their analytical performances.

Although the affinity of the antibody for its antigen may be considered the main factor determining the sensitivity of immunoassays, the question is far more complex. The overall design of ELISAs and LFIAs relies on a stepwise addition of "layers,"

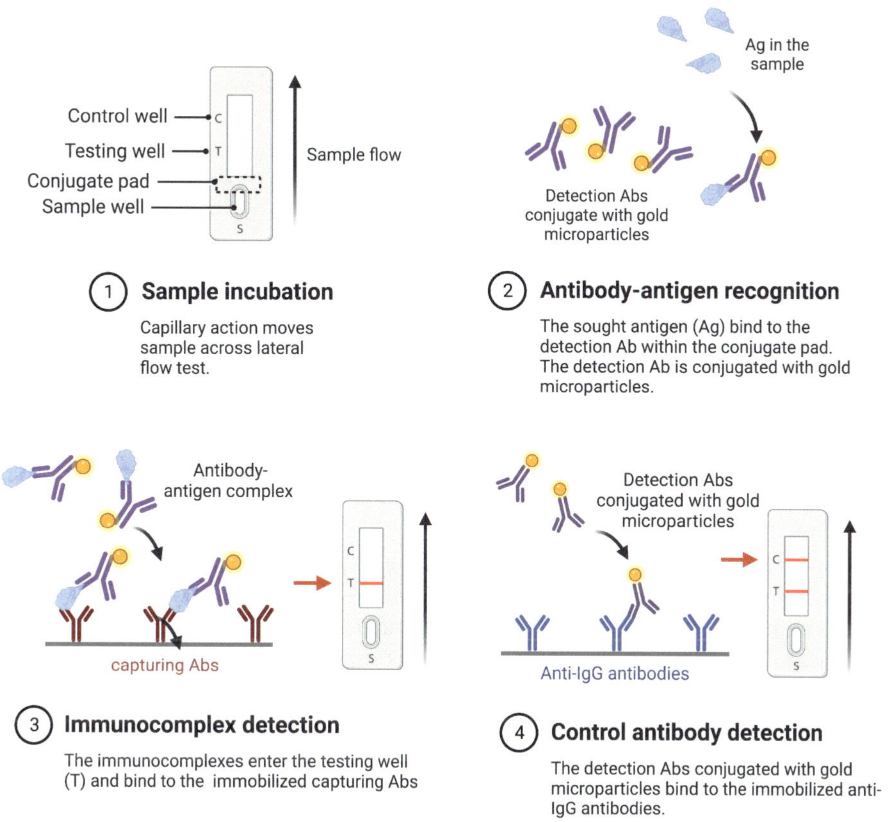

Figure 2.
Representation of the working principle of LFIA.

where each one affects the performance of the following one. Indeed, the type of surfaces, the distribution of Abs, and the physicochemical properties of Ags contribute to determining the analytical performances of immunoassays.

The aim of this chapter is to describe the importance of these features in the development of ELISAs and LFIAs.

2. Antibodies adsorption

ELISA is particularly useful when testing for low levels of analytes in biological samples since the antigen is concentrated by the antibody, which coats the solid surface. Since 90s, researchers have studied how antibodies interact with different plastic surfaces to obtain an efficient binding of the antigen. Stevens and coworkers investigated the adsorption of antibodies on several types of polystyrene microtiter plates with different protein binding capacities [7]. The authors observed two possible patterns of binding. The first followed the Langmuir model, according to which Abs were adsorbed as a monolayer without lateral interactions among them. The second pattern, instead, was characterized by the presence of Ab-Ab interactions. Interestingly, Abs coated according to the second pattern were more susceptible to desorption in the subsequent steps of the ELISA. This could be due to a supersaturating concentration of coated antibodies resulting in the formation of protein multilayers, which are less stable than protein adsorbed directly on hydrophobic surfaces of polystyrene [8, 9]. Therefore, it is recommended the choice of surface materials that allow the formation of Ab monolayers.

Several researchers studied the Abs adsorption on planar surfaces with the aim to describe their distribution and orientation in monolayers. When adsorbed on polystyrene surfaces, Abs can assume four different orientations: end-on (Fab-up or Fab-down), side-on, or flat-on (**Figure 3**).

Buijs and coworkers [10] established the mass of Ab monolayers composed of only one of the possible orientations. The flat-on orientation allowed the binding of 200 ng/cm^2 Abs and the end-on orientation of 370 ng/cm^2 or 550 ng/cm^2, depending on the distance between fragment antigen-binding regions (Fabs). Quartz crystal microbalance measurements showed that monolayers obtained on planar polystyrene by random adsorption contained 468 ng/cm^2 Abs. This value corresponded to a mixture of antibodies orientations, in fact, Abs are initially adsorbed in a flat-on orientation, then the residual binding sites are filled up by Abs in an end-on orientation [11–14].

Several studies showed that the formation of an Ab monolayer depends on the concentration of the solution used to coat polystyrene surfaces. The use of coating solutions containing Abs up to 20 μg/ml was associated with a progressive increase of both adsorbed Abs molecules and antigen-binding capacity. Solutions exceeding the 20 μg/ml threshold favored the deposition of Abs in multilayers that negatively affected the antigen-binding capacity of the surface since the access of antigens to the binding sites is limited by steric hindrance [7, 12, 13, 15–18].

The adsorption of molecules to polystyrene surfaces can be mediated by intermolecular attraction forces (i.e., van der Waals forces), hydrophilic bonds (e.g., hydrogen bonds), or hydrophobic interactions. The type of bond predominantly used by proteins depends on the prevalence of hydrophobic or hydrophilic amino acid residues [19]. Based on this, several types of adsorbent polystyrene surfaces have been developed to promote the adsorption of predominantly hydrophobic or hydrophilic proteins. Regarding Abs, their adsorption is maximized on microtiter plates made from polystyrene modified by adding hydrophilic groups. These types of plates favor also more orderly adsorption of Abs through the interaction between the carbohydrate moieties in their Fc fragments and the hydrophilic groups of the polystyrene surfaces [19].

Physical adsorption of Abs was mainly studied on polystyrene surfaces, but the same principles can be extended to other kinds of solid surfaces such as paper and cellulose membranes. In fact, physical adsorption of Abs may occur on these kinds

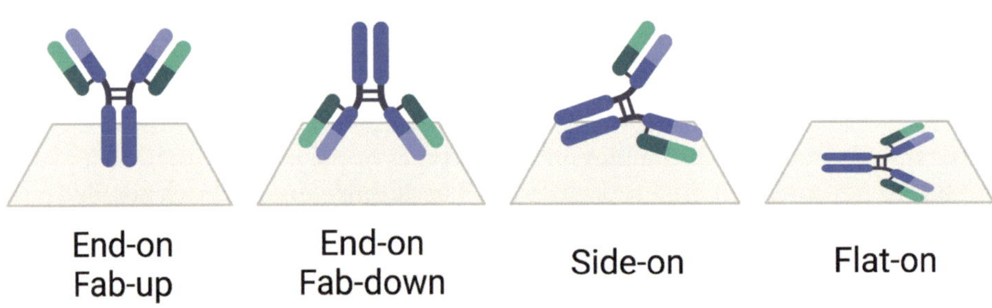

Figure 3.
Different antibodies orientations on polystyrene surface.

of surfaces by van der Waals forces, hydrogen bonds, and hydrophobic interactions. But the leading forces involved in Abs binding on cellulose membrane are the electrostatic interaction between cationic groups of proteins and anionic groups of cellulose itself [20]. Despite the hydrophilic nature of cellulose, also in these cases a partial denaturation and random orientation of Abs have been observed [21, 22]. Currently, researchers are investigating strategies to increase the sensitivity of paper or cellulose-based immunoassays by functionalizing them with suitable chemical compounds to obtain a more homogeneous capturing surface without affecting the folding of Abs. These approaches will be discussed in the next session.

3. Antibodies orientation

As described above, Abs are adsorbed on polystyrene in different orientations that can affect the biological function of Abs. Three out of the four possible orientations (i.e., Fab-down, side-on, or a flat-on) cause the reduction or the loss of antigen-binding capacity [12]. In fact, only 5–10% of the antigen-binding sites are effectively available when Abs are randomly adsorbed on the polystyrene surface [23]. Moreover, the adsorption on polystyrene can induce a partial denaturation of Abs [11, 23–26]. Overall, the spontaneous adsorption of Abs on polystyrene is a widely applied technique due to its ease of use, but it reduces the total antigen-binding capacity of capturing surfaces, and it is associated with a poor signal-to-noise ratio. It is now well established that surfaces coated with Abs uniformly bound in the Fab-up orientation lead to a significant improvement of ELISAs sensitivity. For this reason, several researchers have studied strategies to orient Abs on planar surfaces while preserving their original folding (**Figure 4**).

The first method described to orient Abs is the covalent coupling of their amine or carboxylic groups on chemically activated surfaces [27–31]. This method allowed an improvement in ELISAs sensitivity, but not a uniform distribution of Abs since amino and carboxylic groups are throughout the Ab structure [32]. For this reason, the covalent coupling is not a site-controlled orientation method.

Another approach consisted of the immobilization of Abs based on Ab-biotin/streptavidin-surface complexes that increased the availability of antigen-binding sites up to 70% when Ab was randomly biotinylated [23, 33, 34]. Peluso and coworkers compared the effect of the random or site-direct biotinylation of Abs and Fab fragments on their binding capacity [35]. In this work, Abs were specifically biotinylated on the oligosaccharide moiety of the Fc fragment, while Fab were biotinylated on the reduced thiols of the hinge region. Results showed that site-direct biotinylation of Abs and Fab' provided 10- and 5-fold higher signals, respectively, in comparison with the randomly biotinylated counterpart. As a result of these observations, several site-direct methods to orient Abs have been developed.

A common specific method to orient Abs takes advantage of intermediate proteins that bind the Fc fragment of Abs [36]. Protein A and protein G are cell wall proteins expressed by *Staphylococcus aureus* and *Streptococcus* species, respectively. Both proteins A and G specifically bind amino acid residues at the interface between the constant domains C_{H2} and C_{H3} of mammalian IgGs [37].

Protein A binds all human immunoglobulin G (IgG) subclasses except for IgG3. It can also bind human IgA, IgM, IgE, and mouse IgG2a, IgG2b, and IgG3 [38]. Protein G recognizes Fc domains of all human IgG subclasses, as well as rabbit, mouse, and goat IgGs [39].

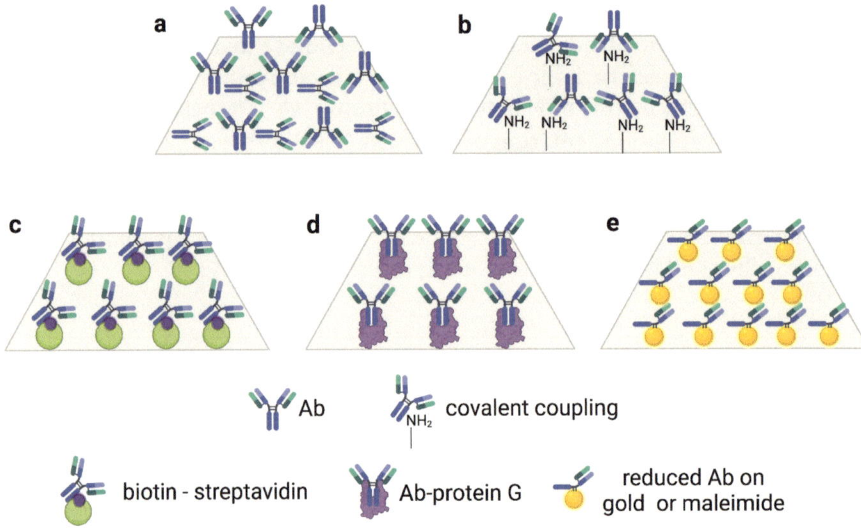

Figure 4.
Antibodies orientation strategies on polystyrene surface. a) Random orientation by adsorption. b) Random orientation by covalent coupling. c) Site-direct orientation by biotinylated antibody and streptavidin-coated surface. d) Site-direct orientation by protein G-coated surface. e) Site-direct orientation by reduced ab on gold or maleimide surface.

Protein G/A were first used in affinity chromatography to purify Abs [40], then their use was extended to immunoassays applications. The first described application was a biosensor for human IgGs detection based on protein A and quartz crystal microbalance [41]. This approach was then applied by Prusak-Sochaczewski and Luong, that described the use of protein A for Ab immobilization in immunoassays [42]. Since then, a number of immunoassays that use protein A/G to orient Abs on the surface were developed; for extensive review elsewhere [43, 44]. It could be argued that also the orientation of protein A/G might affect the overall binding capacity of capturing surface. Orientation of protein A/G affects the Ab density, but experimental results showed that the maximum increase in antigen-binding capacity was obtained with non-oriented protein G/A-Ab complexes compared to randomly adsorbed Ab. Protein A/G orientation did not provide a further significant increase [43].

Another interesting method of site-directed Ab immobilization involves disulfide bridges located in the hinge region of Abs. These disulfide bridges can be specifically reduced by mild reducing agents, such as tris(2-carboxyethyl)phosphine hydrochloride (TCEP), dithiothreitol (DTT), or 2-mercaptoethanolamine (2-MEA). The so-obtained monovalent Abs can self-assemble and spontaneously orient on conveniently functionalized surfaces [45–49]. The functionalization of surfaces includes the layering of gold [50], maleimides [51], and pyridyl disulfides [52]. ELISAs, performed with oriented monovalent antibodies, showed improved antigen-binding capacity compared to the same assay performed with randomly adsorbed Abs [53].

The contribution of reduction and orientation on the antigen-binding capacity was investigated separately by coating monovalent and whole Abs on polystyrene or maleimide functionalized microplates. Results highlighted that the chemical reduction by itself increased the antigen-binding capacity of Abs, probably as a consequence of folding rearrangements that influence the affinity for the antigen-binding site. Orientation was shown to improve both the sensitivity and the reproducibility of the results likely providing a more homogeneous capturing surface [54].

DOI: http://dx.doi.org/10.5772/intechopen.1001374

Some of the approaches previously described to orient Abs on ELISA surfaces have now been applied also to LFIAs to improve their sensitivity. Capturing Abs on the test line (**Figure 2**) can be oriented by using fusion proteins that have a binding site both for cellulose and Fc fragments of Abs. Yang and coworkers [21] developed a fusion protein composed of a cellulose-binding module and the Fc-binding domain of protein A. Authors found that the orientation of capturing Abs on the test line, obtained by the developed fusion protein, increases the sensitivity of the LFIAs when compared to randomly adsorbed Abs [21]. Another interesting approach involves the orientation of the detection Abs instead of the capturing ones. It was shown that also the orientation of Abs on the detection beads increased the sensitivity of the assay and this increase was obtained even if the amount of immobilized Abs was lower in comparison with a random absorption on the beads [55, 56].

To conclude, orientation of Abs increases the overall antigen-binding capacity of ELISA and LFIA surfaces and this contributes to enhance the sensitivity of these kinds of assays. This is especially true for small antigens that have a Stoke radius smaller than those of Abs since, in this case, the simultaneous binding of two antigens for Ab molecule is possible [35].

The contribution of analyte and antibody properties to the sensitivity of oriented ELISAs is discussed in the next section.

4. Effects of antibody and antigen properties on the sensitivity of immunoassays

In the development of immunoassays, one of the key steps is the selection of the Ab to be immobilized on the surface. In this regard, the two factors certainly taken into consideration are the specificity toward the Ag of interest and the affinity constant of the Ab for the selected epitope on the Ag. Anyway, the orientation of the Ab, its avidity, and the physicochemical characteristics of the antigens (size, mono-multivalency) should be also considered.

The importance of Ag properties on the effect of uniform orientation of Abs has been investigated by a few authors. Trilling and coworkers [57] studied how the dimension of Ags affects the sensitivity of ELISAs based on oriented Abs. Considering the Stoke radius of Ags, the authors showed that the greatest advantage in using oriented ELISAs was observed with small Ags, since they could interact with all the accessible antigen-binding sites. Whereas oriented ELISAs for large Ags did not allow for a significant increase in sensitivity in comparison with the non-oriented counterpart. This is probably due to the steric hindrance of Ags that limits access to neighboring antigen-binding sites. These results find confirmation in publications by other researchers [35, 54].

Studies aimed to investigate oriented ELISAs analytical performances in the presence of different concentrations of Ags revealed the importance of considering the affinity of Ab in the setup of ELISAs. The affinity of an Ab for its Ag can be described by the dissociation constant which is a measure of the strength of the interaction between an epitope and a single antigen-binding site. Collected data suggested that affinity is a major determinant of the analytical sensitivity of all types of ELISAs [57], especially in the oriented ELISAs in which the maximum advantage was observed for Ag concentration below the dissociation constant [35, 58].

Avidity is a measure of the overall strength of binding of Ab-Ag complexes, and it depends on the affinity and valency of both Abs and Ags. The role of avidity is especially evident with multimeric Ags, which can engage multiple antigen-binding sites by the repeated epitopes exposed on their surface. The multiple binding leads to the stabilization of the Ab-Ag complexes, suggesting that avidity is the leading force involved in the binding of multimeric Ags. This occurs in both oriented and non-oriented ELISAs [59, 60]. A clue to the role of affinity and avidity on the analytical sensitivity of ELISAs was obtained by comparing a non-oriented and an oriented ELISA for ferritin, a multimeric protein. The same capturing Ab was used for the two assays: in the non-oriented assay polystyrene was coated with whole Ab, while in the oriented assay reduced monovalent Ab was used. As mentioned above, chemical reduction improves the affinity of the antigen-binding site [54]. No differences were observed between the two types of ELISAs for ferritin. These data suggested that the avidity is predominant in affinity when considering multimeric Ags [58].

In light of the described studies, it is possible to conclude that Ag properties, such as dimension and valency, have an important role in the setup of ELISAs, and for extension also in the setup of LFIAs.

5. Conclusions

The formation of the Ab-Ag immunocomplex is one of the factors determining the sensitivity of ELISAs and LFIAs. Its formation is dependent both on the orientation and density of Abs coated on the surface and Ags properties. In ELISAs, the selected polystyrene and the concentration of the Abs coating solution should ensure the formation of a monolayer of Abs in which each Ab molecule interacts directly with the surface. This is the condition that ensures the maximum stability of the binding between Abs and polystyrene but not the maximum accessibility of antigen binding sites. The direct interaction with the surface (polystyrene, paper, or cellulose membrane) can cause a partial denaturation of Abs and the random orientation can mask an unpredictable amount of antigen binding sites. Indeed, it was estimated that only 5–10% of the antigen-binding sites remain effectively available.

To overcome these limits, several strategies have been developed to preserve Abs folding and to orient them with their antigen-binding sites facing outwards the surface. These strategies showed to be efficient in enhancing the sensitivity of ELISAs and LFIAs, besides, studies to develop them stand out the importance of Ags characteristics in determining the formation of Ab-Ag complexes. It can be easily understood that the quantification of small Ags takes advantage of the orientation of Abs as small Ags can effectively use the greater number of accessible antigen-binding sites provided by orientation. It is not so clear the role of the Abs coated surface on the binding of multivalent Ags that can engage multiple antigen-binding sites. Thus, the main property of Abs contributing to the formation of Ab-Ag complexes is avidity, which is often overlooked.

In conclusion, a broader perspective that goes beyond the selection of Abs just on the basis of affinity should be introduced in ELISAs and LFIAs development. Indeed, the best solution to favor the antigen-binding event should be tailored to both the Abs and Ags properties.

Conflict of interest

The authors declare that they have no known competing financial interest or personal relationships that could have appeared to influence the work reported in this paper.

DOI: http://dx.doi.org/10.5772/intechopen.1001374

Author details

Vanessa Susini*, Chiara Sanguinetti, Silvia Ursino, Laura Caponi and Maria Franzini
Department of Translational Research and of New Surgical and Medical Technologies, University of Pisa, Pisa, Italy

*Address all correspondence to: vanessa.susini@med.unipi.it

References

[1] He J. Chapter 5.1 - practical guide to ELISA development. In: Wild D, editor. Immunoass. Handb. Fourth ed. Oxford: Elsevier; 2013. pp. 381-393. DOI: 10.1016/B978-0-08-097037-0.00025-7

[2] Jordan W. Dual-antibody Sandwich enzyme-linked immunosorbent assay. In: Burns R, editor. Immunochem. Protoc. Totowa, NJ: Humana Press; 2005. pp. 207-214. DOI: 10.1385/1-59259-873-0:207

[3] Wilson K, Walker J, editors. Principles and Techniques of Biochemistry and Molecular Biology. 6th ed. Cambridge: Cambridge University Press; 2005. DOI: 10.1017/CBO9780511813412

[4] Engvall E, Perlmann P. Enzyme-linked immunosorbent assay (ELISA). Quantitative assay of immunoglobulin G, Immunochemistry. 1971;**8**:871-874. DOI: 10.1016/0019-2791(71)90454-x

[5] Koczula KM, Gallotta A. Lateral flow assays. Essays in Biochemistry. 2016;**60**:111. DOI: 10.1042/EBC20150012

[6] Di Nardo F, Chiarello M, Cavalera S, Baggiani C, Anfossi L. Ten years of lateral flow immunoassay technique applications: Trends. Challenges and Future Perspectives, Sensors. 2021;**21**:5185. DOI: 10.3390/s21155185

[7] Stevens PW, Hansberry MR, Kelso DM. Assessment of adsorption and adhesion of proteins to polystyrene microwells by sequential enzyme-linked immunosorbent assay analysis. Analytical Biochemistry. 1995;**225**:197-205. DOI: 10.1006/abio.1995.1144

[8] Butler JE. Solid supports in enzyme-linked immunosorbent assay and other solid-phase immunoassays. Methods. 2000;**22**:4-23. DOI: 10.1006/meth.2000.1031

[9] Butler JE, Lü EP, Navarro P, Christiansen B. Comparative studies on the interaction of proteins with a polydimethylsiloxane elastomer. I. Monolayer protein capture capacity (PCC) as a function of protein pl, buffer pH and buffer ionic strength. Journal of Molecular Recognition. 1997;**10**:36-51. DOI: 10.1002/(SICI)1099-1352(199701/02)10:1<36::AID-JMR353>3.0.CO;2-G

[10] Buijs J, Lichtenbelt JWT, Norde W, Lyklema J. Adsorption of monoclonal IgGs and their F(ab′)2 fragments onto polymeric surfaces. Colloids and Surfaces. B, Biointerfaces. 1995;**5**:11-23. DOI: 10.1016/0927-7765(95)98205-2

[11] Wang X, Wang Y, Xu H, Shan H, Lu JR. Dynamic adsorption of monoclonal antibody layers on hydrophilic silica surface: A combined study by spectroscopic ellipsometry and AFM. Journal of Colloid and Interface Science. 2008;**323**:18-25. DOI: 10.1016/j.jcis.2008.04.024

[12] Wiseman ME, Frank CW. Antibody adsorption and orientation on hydrophobic surfaces. Langmuir: the ACS Journal of Surfaces and Colloids. 2012;**28**:1765-1774. DOI: 10.1021/la203095p

[13] Xu H, Zhao X, Grant C, Lu JR, Williams DE, Penfold J. Orientation of a monoclonal antibody adsorbed at the solid/solution Interface: A combined study using atomic force microscopy and neutron reflectivity. Langmuir. 2006;**22**:6313-6320. DOI: 10.1021/la0532454

[14] Zhao X, Pan F, Lu JR. Interfacial assembly of proteins and peptides:

Recent examples studied by neutron reflection. Journal of the Royal Society Interface. 2009;**6**:S659-S670. DOI: 10.1098/rsif.2009.0168.focus

[15] Chen H, Huang J, Lee J, Hwang S, Koh K. Surface plasmon resonance spectroscopic characterization of antibody orientation and activity on the calixarene monolayer. Sensors Actuators, B: Chemistry. 2010;**147**:548-553. DOI: 10.1016/j.snb.2010.03.033

[16] Le NCH, Gubala V, Gandhiraman RP, Coyle C, Daniels S, Williams DE. Total internal reflection ellipsometry as a label-free assessment method for optimization of the reactive surface of bioassay devices based on a functionalized cycloolefin polymer. Analytical and Bioanalytical Chemistry. 2010;**398**:1927-1936. DOI: 10.1007/s00216-010-4099-4

[17] Yuan W, Dong H, Li CM, Cui X, Yu L, Lu Z, et al. pH-controlled construction of chitosan/alginate multilayer film: Characterization and application for antibody immobilization. Langmuir. 2007;**23**:13046-13052. DOI: 10.1021/la702774a

[18] Zhao X, Pan F, Cowsill B, Lu JR, Garcia-Gancedo L, Flewitt AJ, et al. Interfacial immobilization of monoclonal antibody and detection of human prostate-specific antigen. Langmuir. 2011;**27**:7654-7662. DOI: 10.1021/la201245q

[19] Esser P. Principles in Adsorption to Polystyrene. Thermo Scientific Application Note. 2014. Available from: https://assets.thermofisher.com/TFS-Assets/LSG/Application-Notes/D19559.pdf

[20] Kong F, Hu YF. Biomolecule immobilization techniques for bioactive paper fabrication. Analytical and Bioanalytical Chemistry. 2012;**403**:7-13. DOI: 10.1007/s00216-012-5821-1

[21] Yang JM, Kim KR, Jeon S, Cha HJ, Kim CS. A sensitive paper-based lateral flow immunoassay platform using engineered cellulose-binding protein linker fused with antibody-binding domains. Sensors Actuators, B: Chemistry. 2021;**329**:129099. DOI: 10.1016/j.snb.2020.129099

[22] Zhu H, Snyder M. Protein chip technology. Current Opinion in Chemical Biology. 2003;**7**:55-63. DOI: 10.1016/S1367-5931(02)00005-4

[23] Butler JE, Ni L, Nessler R, Joshi KS, Suter M, Rosenberg B, et al. The physical and functional behavior of capture antibodies adsorbed on polystyrene. Journal of Immunological Methods. 1992;**150**:77-90. DOI: 10.1016/0022-1759(92)90066-3

[24] Ball V, Huetz P, Elaissari A, Cazenave JP, Voegel JC, Schaaf P. Kinetics of exchange processes in the adsorption of proteins on solid surfaces. Proceedings of the National Academy of Sciences. 1994;**91**:7330-7334. DOI: 10.1073/pnas.91.15.7330

[25] Butler JE, Ni L, Brown WR, Joshi KS, Chang J, Rosenberg B, et al. The immunochemistry of sandwich ELISAs--VI. Greater than 90% of monoclonal and 75% of polyclonal anti-fluorescyl capture antibodies (CAbs) are denatured by passive adsorption. Molecular Immunology. 1993;**30**:1165-1175. DOI: 10.1016/0161-5890(93)90135-x

[26] Huetz P, Ball V, Voegel J-C, Schaaf P. Exchange kinetics for a heterogeneous protein system on a solid surface. Langmuir. 1995;**11**:3145-3152. DOI: 10.1021/la00008a046

[27] Dixit CK, Vashist SK, MacCraith BD, O'Kennedy R. Multisubstrate-compatible ELISA procedures for rapid and high-sensitivity immunoassays. Nature

Protocols. 2011;**6**:439-445. DOI: 10.1038/nprot.2011.304

[28] Bin L, Xie J, Lu C, Wu C, Wei Y. Oriented immobilization of fab' fragments on silica surfaces. Analytical Chemistry. 1995;**67**:83-87. DOI: 10.1021/ac00097a014

[29] Nakanishi K, Muguruma H, Karube I. A novel method of immobilizing antibodies on a quartz crystal microbalance using plasma-polymerized films for immunosensors. Analytical Chemistry. 1996;**68**:1695-1700. DOI: 10.1021/ac950756u

[30] Spitznagel TM, Clark DS. Surface-density and orientation effects on immobilized antibodies and antibody fragments. Bio/Technology. 1993;**11**:825-829. DOI: 10.1038/nbt0793-825

[31] Vijayendran RA, Leckband DE. A quantitative assessment of heterogeneity for surface-immobilized proteins. Analytical Chemistry. 2001;**73**:471-480. DOI: 10.1021/ac000523p

[32] Goddard JM, Hotchkiss JH. Polymer surface modification for the attachment of bioactive compounds. Progress in Polymer Science. 2007;**32**:698-725. DOI: 10.1016/j.progpolymsci.2007.04.002

[33] Morgan H, Taylor DM. A surface plasmon resonance immunosensor based on the streptavidin-biotin complex. Biosensors & Bioelectronics. 1992;**7**:405-410. DOI: 10.1016/0956-5663(92)85039-d

[34] Rowe CA, Scruggs SB, Feldstein MJ, Golden JP, Ligler FS. An array immunosensor for simultaneous detection of clinical analytes. Analytical Chemistry. 1999;**71**:433-439. DOI: 10.1021/ac980798t

[35] Peluso P, Wilson DS, Do D, Tran H, Venkatasubbaiah M, Quincy D, et al. Optimizing antibody immobilization strategies for the construction of protein microarrays. Analytical Biochemistry. 2003;**312**:113-124. DOI: 10.1016/s0003-2697(02)00442-6

[36] Sauer-Eriksson AE, Kleywegt GJ, Uhlén M, Jones TA. Crystal structure of the C2 fragment of streptococcal protein G in complex with the fc domain of human IgG. Structure. 1995;**3**:265-278. DOI: 10.1016/S0969-2126(01)00157-5

[37] Deisenhofer J. Crystallographic refinement and atomic models of a human fc fragment and its complex with fragment B of protein a from Staphylococcus aureus at 2.9- and 2.8-Å resolution. Biochemistry. 1981;**20**:2361-2370. DOI: 10.1021/bi00512a001

[38] Surolia A, Pain D, Islam Khan M. Protein a: nature's universal anti-antibody. Trends in Biochemical Sciences. 1982;**7**:74-76. DOI: 10.1016/0968-0004(82)90082-2

[39] Bjorck L, Kronvall G. Purification and some properties of streptococcal protein G, a novel IgG-binding reagent. Journal of Immunology. 1984;**133**:969-974

[40] Bürckstümmer T, Bennett KL, Preradovic A, Schütze G, Hantschel O, Superti-Furga G, et al. An efficient tandem affinity purification procedure for interaction proteomics in mammalian cells. Nature Methods. 2006;**3**:1013-1019. DOI: 10.1038/nmeth968

[41] Muramatsu H, Dicks JM, Tamiya E, Karube I. Piezoelectric crystal biosensor modified with protein a for determination of immunoglobulins. Analytical Chemistry. 1987;**59**:2760-2763. DOI: 10.1021/ac00150a007

[42] Prusak-Sochaczewski E, Luong JHT. A new approach to the development of a

reusable piezoelectric crystal biosensor. Analytical Letters. 1990;**23**:401-409. DOI: 10.1080/00032719008052452

[43] Makaraviciute A, Ramanaviciene A. Site-directed antibody immobilization techniques for immunosensors. Biosensors & Bioelectronics. 2013;**50**:460-471. DOI: 10.1016/j.bios.2013.06.060

[44] Shen M, Rusling J, Dixit CK. Site-selective orientated immobilization of antibodies and conjugates for immunodiagnostics development. Methods San Diego California. 2017;**116**:95-111. DOI: 10.1016/j.ymeth.2016.11.010

[45] Balevicius Z, Ramanaviciene A, BaleviciuteI,MakaraviciuteA,MikoliunaiteL, Ramanavicius A. Evaluation of intact- and fragmented-antibody based immunosensors by total internal reflection ellipsometry. Sensors and Actuators, B: Chemistry. 2011;**160**:555-562. DOI: 10.1016/j.snb.2011.08.029

[46] Baleviciute I, Balevicius Z, Makaraviciute A, Ramanaviciene A, Ramanavicius A. Study of antibody/antigen binding kinetics by total internal reflection ellipsometry. Biosensors & Bioelectronics. 2013;**39**:170-176. DOI: 10.1016/j.bios.2012.07.017

[47] Baniukevic J, Hakki Boyaci I, Goktug Bozkurt A, Tamer U, Ramanavicius A, Ramanaviciene A. Magnetic gold nanoparticles in SERS-based sandwich immunoassay for antigen detection by well oriented antibodies. Biosensors & Bioelectronics. 2013;**43**:281-288. DOI: 10.1016/j.bios.2012.12.014

[48] Hermanson GT. Chapter 2 - functional targets for bioconjugation. In: Hermanson GT, editor. Bioconjugate Tech. Third ed. Boston: Academic Press; 2013. pp. 127-228. DOI: 10.1016/B978-0-12-382239-0.00002-9

[49] Ho JAA, Hsu W-L, Liao W-C, Chiu J-K, Chen M-L, Chang H-C, et al. Ultrasensitive electrochemical detection of biotin using electrically addressable site-oriented antibody immobilization approach via aminophenyl boronic acid. Biosensors & Bioelectronics. 2010;**26**:1021-1027. DOI: 10.1016/j.bios.2010.08.048

[50] Dixit CK, Kumar A, Kaushik A. Nanosphere lithography-based platform for developing rapid and high sensitivity microarray systems. Biochemical and Biophysical Research Communications. 2012;**423**:473-477. DOI: 10.1016/j.bbrc.2012.05.144

[51] Billah MM, Hodges CS, Hays HCW, Millner PA. Directed immobilization of reduced antibody fragments onto a novel SAM on gold for myoglobin impedance immunosensing. Bioelectrochemistry Amsterdam, Netherlands. 2010;**80**:49-54. DOI: 10.1016/j.bioelechem.2010.08.005

[52] Iwasaki Y, Omichi Y, Iwata R. Site-specific dense immobilization of antibody fragments on polymer brushes supported by silicone nanofilaments. Langmuir: the ACS Journal of Surfaces Colloids. 2008;**24**:8427-8430. DOI: 10.1021/la801327a

[53] Kausaite-Minkstimiene A, Ramanaviciene A, Kirlyte J, Ramanavicius A. Comparative study of random and oriented antibody immobilization techniques on the binding capacity of immunosensor. Analytical Chemistry. 2010;**82**:6401-6408. DOI: 10.1021/ac100468k

[54] Susini V, Caponi L, Rossi VL, Sanesi A, Romiti N, Paolicchi A, et al. Sensitivity and reproducibility enhancement in enzyme immunosorbent assays based on half fragment antibodies. Analytical Biochemistry. 2020;**616**:114090. DOI: 10.1016/j.ab.2020.114090

[55] Ryu Y, Jin Z, Kang MS, Kim H-S. Increase in the detection sensitivity of a lateral flow assay for a cardiac marker by oriented immobilization of antibody. BioChip Journal. 2011;**5**:193-198. DOI: 10.1007/s13206-011-5301-2

[56] Lou D, Fan L, Cui Y, Zhu Y, Gu N, Zhang Y. Fluorescent Nanoprobes with oriented modified antibodies to improve lateral flow immunoassay of cardiac troponin I. Analytical Chemistry. 2018;**90**:6502-6508. DOI: 10.1021/acs.analchem.7b05410

[57] Trilling AK, Harmsen MM, Ruigrok VJB, Zuilhof H, Beekwilder J. The effect of uniform capture molecule orientation on biosensor sensitivity: Dependence on analyte properties. Biosensors & Bioelectronics. 2013;**40**:219-226. DOI: 10.1016/j.bios.2012.07.027

[58] Susini V, Fierabracci V, Barria G, Dodoli L, Caponi L, Paolicchi A, et al. Signal enhancement in oriented immunosorbent assays: A balance between accessibility of antigen binding sites and avidity. Biosensors. 2021;**11**:493. DOI: 10.3390/bios11120493

[59] Bush DB, Knotts TA. The effects of antigen size, binding site valency, and flexibility on fab-antigen binding near solid surfaces. The Journal of Chemical Physics. 2018;**149**:165102. DOI: 10.1063/1.5045356

[60] Pukin AV, Branderhorst HM, Sisu C, Weijers CAGM, Gilbert M, Liskamp RMJ, et al. Strong inhibition of cholera toxin by multivalent GM1 derivatives. Chembiochem. 2007;**8**:1500-1503. DOI: 10.1002/cbic.200700266

Chapter 8

Nanobody Technology and New Molecular Biology Methods to Advance Rapid Diagnostic Test for Neglected Tropical Diseases

Andrés Álvarez-Rodríguez, Magdalena Radwanska, Stefan Magez and Steven Odongo

Abstract

Worldwide, the cumulative annual disabilities and deaths due to neglected tropical diseases (NTDs) are in the millions, with most cases found in the low-income countries. The World Health Organization (WHO) has proposed a road map to eliminate NTDs by the year 2030. Core interventions being implemented to achieve this target are vaccinations, chemotherapeutic treatments, vector control, and practicing hygiene. Whereas multiple successes have been registered so far, inadequacies or the complete absence of diagnostics for some of the diseases being targeted, are however hampering ongoing eradication campaigns. Current diagnostics for NTDs are costly, require sophisticated gadgets, depend on electricity, are time consuming and labor intensive, have low detection/discriminatory power, or require trained personnel for operation. For these reasons, the use of such diagnostics is limited to only well-equipped laboratories, often inaccessible to the poor who are the most affected by the NTDs. To increase accessibility to diagnostics by those who need it the most, Rapid Diagnostic Tests (RDTs) are being developed by translating existing diagnostic technologies, or by invention of new technologies. Here, we reviewed conventional diagnostics for NTDs as well as their RDT translated formats, and explored nanobodies (Nbs) as alternative reagents for the development of the RDTs.

Keywords: nanobodies, rapid antigen test, diagnosis, neglected tropical diseases, molecular biology

1. Introduction

According to data from the WHO, communicable diseases ranked among the top 10 causes of deaths in the low-income countries [1]. In contrast, high-income countries control these diseases through vigorous implementation of prevention and treatment campaigns, reinforced with timely diagnosis. Recently, the WHO has established a road map for eradication of the neglected tropical diseases NTDs, by the year 2030 [2]. Neglected tropical diseases are designated as "neglected" partly because

 IntechOpen

they are frequently overlooked by health systems [2]. They include buruli ulcers, chagas disease, dengue, and chikungunya, dracunculiasis, echinococcosis, foodborne trematodiases (FBT), Human African trypanosomiasis (HAT), leishmaniasis, leprosy, lymphatic filariasis, mycetoma/chromoblastomycosis and other deep mycoses, onchocerciasis, rabies, scabies and other ectoparasitoses, schistosomiasis, soil-transmitted helminthiases (STH), snakebite envenoming, taeniasis and cysticercosis, trachoma, and yaws. A foreseen set-back to the WHO's 2030 road map to elimination of NTDs, is the inadequate deployment of diagnostics for case finding, treatment follow-up, and surveillance. It should be noted that even COVID-19 test is not widely accessible, which has left the population in a precarious state.

The conventional methods for diagnosis of NTDs can be classified into eight groups: (i) nucleic acid amplification tests (NAATs), methods for detection of whole or part of a pathogen genome; (ii) immunoassays, methods for detection of a pathogen antigenic (Ag) component, or a pathogen-induced host antibodies (Abs); (iii) microscopy, methods for detection of a pathogen, or its pathological effect(s); (iv) culture, methods for isolating pathogen from clinical specimen using either in vitro or in vivo culture systems followed by either direct or indirect detection with other tests, or detection based on growth characteristics; (v) imaging, non-invasive visual methods for revealing a pathogen or gross deformities caused by a pathogen that are located in situ; (vi) chemical profiling, methods for analyzing chemical components and/or characteristics of a pathogen; (vii) entomological identification, methods for tracking a pathogen in its arthropod vector sentinel for human infections; and (viii) clinical manifestation, methods for detection of a pathogen by drawing inference from the accompanying pathognomonic behavioral changes and/or gross lesions. Each of these methods of diagnosis is further expounded in Section 2.1. Except for the clinical sign-based diagnosis, methods that rely on laboratory testing are not widely applied in impoverished communities due to high costs, absence of well-equipped laboratories, absence of electricity, lack of professionally trained machine operators and maintenance personnel, and complexities surrounding interpretation of assay results. To overcome the listed challenges, modifications of the conventional laboratory-based diagnostic tools and methods are needed. Such modifications include (i) miniaturization, (ii) elimination of multiple assay steps, (iii) multiplexing, and (iv) visual interpretation applications. Nowadays there are simplified diagnostic technologies with enhanced speed, popularly known as RDTs. Given that RDTs have led to effective management of malaria, tuberculosis, and HIV/AIDS in low-income countries, their integration in the NTD control panels is anticipated to yield a positive outcome.

While several authors have reported development of RDT prototypes for NTDs, only a few are so far being marketed [3]. One of the reasons for this is the technical limitations encountered by relatively low sensitivity and specificity. While antigen detecting diagnostics are specific with respect to their capacity to report active infection [4, 5], they usually have low sensitivity, especially when the pathogen load is low or immune complexes between target antigens and infection induced host antibodies are formed [6]. To tackle this, there is ongoing exploratory research involving the use of Nbs [7]. The invention of nanobody technology dates to the year 1993, when Hamers-Casterman et al. discovered heavy-chain only IgG antibodies (HCAbs) in the serum of *Camelus dromedarius* [8]. In the recent past, the application of Nb technology for the development of antigen detection RDTs for infectious diseases have tremendously increased [9–11], exploiting unique epitopes recognition potential of Nbs [12, 13]. Given that Nb epitopes can be located in 'pockets', such as invariant enzyme active sites, their use can ameliorate false negative test resulting from variant natures of surface exposed epitopes [14]. A second advantage of Nb technology is that due to the recombinant production of these molecules, they can easily be tailored [7]. These characteristics allow for Nbs to be used for the development of accessible, sensitive, and specific antigen RDTs.

In this chapter, we reviewed available diagnostics for NTDs focusing on conventional as well as commercialized RDTs and the ongoing efforts to develop rapid antigen RDT using Nbs.

2. Conventional methods for diagnosis of neglected tropical diseases

A plethora of diagnostic platforms are applied singly, or in combination, to achieve diagnosis of NTDs. In principle, each of the conventional diagnostic platforms is multi-spectrum based, being used for the detection of more than one NTD. There are circumstances where modifications were introduced to conventional diagnostics, yielding versions with higher sensitivities and specificities. While these newer versions may have better performance, some have become too complex, rendering them ineffective for field use. As earlier mentioned, most of these diagnostics do not operate as an entity but complement each other. In this section, therefore, the different classical diagnostic methods used either for screening or confirming NTDs, including their modified versions, are reviewed.

2.1 Nucleic acid amplification tests

Nearly 90% of the NTDs are diagnosed by nucleic acid amplification test (NAAT) methods (**Table 1**). The first-generation NAAT technology, the polymerase chain reaction (PCR), was invented in 1983 by Kary Mullis [15]. At present, PCR technology is widely applied in diagnosis and other fields of biosciences. The technology is used for diagnosis of NTDs including Buruli ulcers [16], Dengue [17], Chikungunya [18], HAT [19], leishmaniasis [20], Dracunculiasis [21], deep mycoses [22], onchocerciasis [23], rabies [24], STH [25], and yaws [26] among others. PCR lends itself as a sensitive pathogen detection tool owing to its ability to amplify a single copy of genome to billions of copies. The diagnostic scope of the original PCR was broadened by introducing several modifications. Popular versions of PCR used for diagnosis of NTDs are the reverse transcriptase (RT)-PCR, and real-time RT-PCR. Because it can copy RNA to DNA followed by amplification, RT-PCR is used for diagnosis of the two RNA viral NTDs, i.e., chikungunya [18] and dengue [17]. Real-time RT-PCR, for quantification of nucleic acid load, is used for diagnosis of viral, bacterial, parasitic as well as fungal NTDs. There are groups of pathogens that cannot be discriminated base on NAAT alone, because they have the same amplicon product size. A number of tricks were introduced to solved this challenge, and two examples are given here. Firstly, a second set of nested primers, in a technique call nested PCR, has been introduced to amplify the inner region of the first amplicon product, resulting in variant product sizes. Nested PCR is used for typing the agents for buruli ulcers [16], dengue [17], echinococcosis [27], and HAT [28]. Secondly, a restriction enzyme system, in a technique call restriction fragment length polymorphism (RFLP), was introduced to cut amplified PCR products into fragments producing distinct pathogen-specific restriction profiles. PCR-RFLP technique is used for typing the causative agents of trypanosomiasis [29], leishmaniasis [30], lymphatic filariasis [31] and STH [32].

Conventional Diagnostic Methods	Diagnostic Formats	Neglected topical diseases																				
		Buruli ulcers	Chagas disease	Dengue	Chikungunya	Dracunculiasis	Echinococcosis	FBT	HAT	Leishmaniasis	Leprosy	Lymphatic filariasis	Deep mycoses	Onchocerciasis	Rabies	Ectoparasitoses	Schistosomiasis	STH	Snakebite envenoming	Taeniasis/cysticercosis	Trachoma	Yaws
NAAT	cPCR					+	+	+	+		+	+	+	+			+	+		+	+	+
	RT-PCR			+																		
	nPCR	+		+			+		+													
	rRT-PCR	+	+	+	+			+		+	+	+		+	+							
	PCR-RFLP								+	+	+	+									+	
Immunoassay	ELISA		+	+	+		+	+	+	+	+	+	+	+			+	+		+	+	
	IFA		+		+				+				+		+						+	
	VNT			+											+							
	Hypersensitvity test	+								+	+			+								
	MBA					+																
	WB		+				+			+												
	(Hem)Agglutination Assay		+						+	+							+					+
	HI			+																		
	CFT						+		+													
Microscopy	Unstained smears		+			+	+	+	+		+	+		+		+	+	+		+		
	Stained smears	+	+						+	+											+	+
	Histopathology	+	+							+	+		+		+							+
Culture	*In vitro*	+		+	+					+			+									
	In vivo								+	+	+											

Conventional Diagnostic Methods	Diagnostic Formats	Neglected topical diseases																				
		Buruli ulcers	Chagas disease	Dengue	Chikungunya	Dracunculiasis	Echinococcosis	FBT	HAT	Leishmaniasis	Leprosy	Lymphatic filariasis	Deep mycoses	Onchocerciasis	Rabies	Ectoparasitoses	Schistosomiasis	STH	Snakebite envenoming	Taeniasis/cysticercosis	Trachoma	Yaws
Imagine	Radiography		+			+							+									
	Ultrasonography						+	+					+	+						+		
	MRI						+													+		
	CT scan						+													+		
Chemical profile analyses	MLEE									+												
	MALDI-TOF (MS)								+	+												
	Blood clot test																		+			
Xenodiagnoses	Animals								+													
	Insects								+	+												
Clinical signs	Gross lesions	+				+			+	+	+	+	+	+		+		+	+	+	+	+
	Behavioral														+					+		
Others	Echocardiogram		+																			
	Electrocardiogram		+																			

(1) Symbols: positive-sign (+), diagnostic method is frequently applied for diagnosis of a given NTD; empty box (), scare or no reports showing application of the diagnostic method for diagnosis of that NTD.
(2) Abbreviations: FBT, foodborne trematodiases; HAT, Human African Trypanosomiasis; STH, Soil-transmitted helminths; NAAT, nucleic acid amplification test; PCR, polymerase chain reaction; cPCR, conventional PCR; RT-PCR, Reverse transcriptase PCR; nPCR, Nested PCR; rRT-PCR, real-time reverse transcriptase PCR; PCR-RFLP, PCR restriction fragment length polymorphism; IFA, Immunofluorescence assay; VNT, virus neutralization test; MBA, Multiplex bead assay; WB, Western blot; HI, Hemagglutination inhibition assay; CFT, Complement fixation test; MRI, Magnetic resonance imaging; MLEE, Multilocus Enzyme Electrophoresis; and MALDI-TOF (MS), Matrix assisted laser desorption/ionization time of flight mass spectrometry.

Table 1.
Summary of conventional test platforms used for diagnosis of the neglected tropical diseases.

The NAAT technology revolutionized diagnosis of infectious diseases including NTDs by being robust, high throughput, none labor intensive, sensitive, and specific. Furthermore, NAAT technology allows for multi-pathogen detection through multiplexing [26, 33]. However, with all the desirable qualities, routine mass use of NAAT for diagnosis of NTDs is hampered by costs, its complexity, the requirement for trained operators, and the requirement for expensive equipment as well as a constant supply of electricity. Also, NAAT is sensitive to contaminants, leading to an increased risk for false negative or positive results. Recently introduced among the NAAT-based test panels, is the loop mediated isothermal amplification (LAMP) assay [34]. The LAMP assay has brought NAAT technology closer to its ideal status suitable for routine diagnosis of NTDs in a primary healthcare setting [35, 36]. The LAMP assay is rapid, and it requires less expensive reaction step incubation equipment making it adaptable to field conditions. However, in its current form LAMP is not yet fully furnished to service primary healthcare. At times, the assay still requires sample processing, incurring additional costs and posing contamination risk. The interpretation of LAMP result is subjective, the technique is not completely equipment free, and it still require invasive method of sample collection. Generally, NAAT technology does not yet meet the WHO requirements for an ideal test, which should be Affordable, Sensitive, Specific, User-friendly, Equipment-free and Deliverable to those who need it (ASSURED) [37]. Therefore, further investment is required to produce an ideal NAAT, which is superior to the current version of LAMP assay. Nevertheless, in its current form the LAMP assay has tremendously aided field diagnosis of some NTDs.

2.2 Immunoassays

Immunoassays are well-embedded in the diagnosis of NTDs. Undoubtedly, immunoassays form a large proportion of commercially available NTD diagnostics, and those undergoing development. According the literature reviewed, about 90% of the NTDs are diagnose by immunoassay. Versions of immunoassays exist for laboratory as well as field diagnosis of NTDs. Among others, dengue, chikungunya, echinococcosis, FBT, HAT, leishmaniasis, onchocerciasis, yaws, STH, schistosomiasis, and rabies diagnosis all rely on immunoassays. There are traditional as well as contemporary formats in the NTD diagnostic panels. The most popular classical immunoassay format used for diagnosis of NTDs is the enzyme-linked immunosorbent assay (ELISA). The ELISA technique was published in early 1970's by Van Weemen and Schuurs [38]. This versatile technique is very instrumental in the diagnosis of several NTDs as shown in **Table 1**. As noted previously, ELISA is among those "dual-purpose" immunoassay methods in use either for antibody or antigen detection. Antibody detection ELISAs for diagnosis of NTDs are many but only a few examples are listed here; the Hemagen ELISA for chagas disease [39], MAC-ELISA for dengue [40], Em2-ELISA for echinococcosis [41], the anti-*Mycobacterium leprae* phenolic glycolipid I (PGL-I) IgM ELISA for leprosy [42], the Ov-16 ELISA for onchocerciasis [43], and the FAST-ELISA for schistosomiasis [44]. Unlike antibody detecting ELISA, fewer antigen detecting ELISAs for diagnosis of NTDs exist. An example of antigen detecting ELISA is the CA-ELISA for diagnosis of FBT [45] and Og4C3 ELISA for lymphatic filariasis [46]. Besides ELISA, other popular formats of immunoassay for diagnosis of NTDs are (in)direct immunofluorescence, virus neutralization assays, delayed-type hypersensitivity reaction skin tests, multiplex bead assay, western blot, in(direct) agglutination assays, hemagglutination inhibition assays, and complement fixation assays. Respective NTDs diagnosed by each of these immunoassay formats are listed in **Table 1**.

Like NAAT, classical immunoassay formats do suffer from limitations. In addition to some of the challenges shared with the NAAT, classical immunoassays are low-throughput, labor intensive, and often have lower sensitivity and specificity values. Efforts are underway to translate laboratory-based immunoassay formats to a field applicable point-of-care test (POC), which are suitable for primary health care settings where most of the NTD cases are frequently reported. The commonly encountered POC test frameworks are immunochromatographic test strips, and agglutination assays. The POC test immunoassays have largely solved challenges related to portability and speed. However, the sensitivity and specificity remain often suboptimal. Antibody detection tests, which form the bigger proportion of the current POC immunoassays for NTDs, commonly give false positive test results either due to cross-reactivity [47] or persistence of antibodies after the clearance of infections [48]. False negative test resulting from low pathogen load, sequestration of target in immune complex, and loss of antigen integrity following poor sample handling, characterize most antigen detecting POC tests. All these limitations demand that alternative options are sought to improve the specificity as well as sensitivity of the available immunoassay formats. Hence, this justifies the reason for Nb technology exploration in this area.

2.3 Microscopy

Microscopy is perhaps the most ancient diagnostic platform for the NTDs. The technology was developed by Antony van Leeuwenhoek, a Dutch microbiologist and microscopist, who lived in the fifteenth century in Delft, Holland [49]. For the different models and types of microscopes used for pathogen detection, standard microbiology text books can be consulted such as the *Microbial Life* [49], *Brock Biology of Microorganism* [50], and *Jawetz, Melnick & Adelberg's Medical Microbiology* [51]. Essentially, diagnosis of all the NTDs, except snakebite envenoming, rely on direct or indirect microscopy. Originally the technique relies either on direct visualization of a magnified whole dead (or living) pathogen [52–54], a pathogen product like eggs [55], or a pathogen induced lesions [56]. When used for detection of viral NTDs, microscopy reveals infection-induced cellular changes known as cytopathic effects, such as rabies viral-induced inclusion bodies (Negri bodies) in the cytoplasm of neurons [57]. Dengue fever virus and chikungunya viruses are also detected based on characteristic inclusion bodies, which appear in the in vitro cell cultures.

While microscopy remain a definitive test for some NTDs, poor detection limit often affects its usability. To improve performance, refinements of the methods as well as the tool were made. The modifications introduced to increase resolution power of microscopy for diagnosis of NTDs include the introduction of specimen staining with dyes (e.g., giemsa staining), or by chemical-labeled Abs (immunofluorescence). Thanks to the improvements the acid-fast *Mycobacterium ulcerans*, the agent of buruli ulcer, can now be easily detected upon specimen staining with Ziehl-Neelsen dye, and the rabies virus antigen in brain tissue section can be revealed upon immunofluorescent-labelling with the anti-rabies protein Abs. In other circumstances, the NTD reagent is amplified by growing in an in vivo (animal model) or in vitro (artificial media or cell line) culture system to a high density prior to detection by microscopy. For example, *Trypanosoma* and *Leishmania* are sometimes cultured in mouse model prior to detection by microscopy. Similar, *M. ulcerans*, *M. leprae*, chikungunya, and *actinomycetoma* are sometimes isolated in an in vitro culture system prior to detection. While much as the improvements cited enhance the diagnostic power of microscopy, these refined techniques still require electricity, and are time-consuming and labor intensive. In addition, interpretation of test result is often subjective with low discriminatory power. Integration of pathogen culture with microscopy also exposes assay operators to high-risk pathogens, and there is a possibility of introducing environmental contaminants, which could jeopardize assay results. Finally, advanced microscopes are unsuitable for routine clinical practice, and are limited to research purposes, as they are expensive and complex. Hence, some of the limitations of microscopy cited herein prevent its routine use in a primary healthcare.

2.4 Isolation of pathogen in a culture system

A definitive diagnosis for some the pathogens causing NTDs relies on their amplification in a culture system(s) to attain disease symptoms, or high pathogen density to ease detection [30]. In this instance, interpretation of the result is dependent on phenotypic characteristics including development of pathological changes in an in vitro or in vivo culture system. The cultured organisms may also be subjected to subsidiary confirmatory tests including biochemical assays, microscopy, NAAT, immunoassays among others. The diagnosis of *M. leprae*, for example, is based on culturing the organism, which usually takes up to 14 days. Thereafter, colonial morphologic characteristics are established, and other standard staining techniques, immunoassays and NAAT are implemented for characterization the agent. Culture as a diagnostic test is a long procedure given that it requires multiple steps. Where primary microbiological test results are general, secondary tests are employed to confirm the diagnosis. Pathogen isolation is not only time consuming but it is also prone to errors, which can occur at any of the assay steps. Often expensive materials are required from culturing the organisms until getting the test results subsequently increasing the overall costs of testing. Maintaining sterile conditions for pathogen isolation is huge challenge in the low-income countries. Furthermore, not all the pathogens can be isolated in an artificial in vitro culture system, and ethical issues impede the use of laboratory animals in diagnosis. Although microbiological culture system cannot be avoided altogether, a shift to RDTs would offer solution to some of these challenges.

2.5 Imaging

Imaging is a non-invasive technique for scanning the body of a pathogen or tissue deformities. The technique can be used for diagnosis of several diseases [58]. As tool for diagnosis of NTDs, imaging techniques are commonly applied for diagnosis of dracunculiasis [59], echinococcosis/hydatid cyst [60], FBT [61], onchocerciasis [62], and Taeniasis/neurocysticercosis [63]. The tool is also used for indirect diagnosis of chagas disease by indirectly inferring from the destruction of the myocardium [39]. A collection of imaging technique applied in the diagnosis of NTDs are radiography (employs ionizing radiations like x-rays and gamma rays), ultrasonography, magnetic resonance imaging (MRI), and computerized tomography (CT) scan. Radiography is used for the diagnosis of chagas disease, dracunculiasis, and deep mycoses; ultrasonography for echinococcosis, FBT, deep mycoses, onchocerciasis, and cysticercosis; and both MRI and CT scan for echinococcosis and cysticercosis. Although they may not perfectly fit here, it is worth mentioning that electrocardiogram and echocardiogram are valuable biosensing tools used for diagnosis of chagas disease. Imaging is a preferred technique because it is non-invasive. Routine application of imaging techniques in low resource settings is however impracticable. The most advanced imaging technique requires well-equipped laboratory employing highly qualified personnel for the operation as well as the interpretation of the test result. Additionally, continuous exposure to radioactive materials, which is a fundamental component of radiography, poses health-risks. With the availability of hand-held ultrasonography, the use of imaging is no longer restricted to a laboratory setting. However, the high cost of ultrasonographic equipment impedes it wide scale deployment in a primary healthcare. Miniaturizing the technique while eliminating the cost and complexity would popularize its use in remote settings such as the pastoral communities, where the cysticercosis is highly prevalent.

2.6 Chemical profile analysis

The analysis of the levels of toxins or metabolic by-products deliberately, accidentally, or unintentionally elaborated by foreign organisms into a patient or in the culture system can lead to a diagnosis. On the other hand, aberrant functions of the host's physiological biochemicals such as enzymes and hormones, are sometimes measured during disease investigation process. A few situations standout to exemplify the chemical profiling analysis in disease diagnosis. For instance, the diagnosis of snake bites envenoming relies on coagulopathic tests, which is a 20-minute whole blood clotting test (WBCT20) POC test. There is also a thin layer chromatography tests for detection of *M. ulcerans*, the causative agent of buruli ulcers, which relies on testing for the elaborated mycolactone toxin [64]. Chemical assay tests are less specific, rendering it impossible to target treatment to a specific species or strains causing the disease where species-specific treatment is required. Some of the NTDs are detected based on their signature proteome profiles. Examples in this category are the Multilocus Enzyme Electrophoresis (MLEE) [65], which is used for typing leishmania, and the matrix assisted laser desorption ionization-time of flight-mass spectrometry (MALDI-TOF MS) for leishmania [30] and HAT [66]. The MALDI-TOF and MLEE analyses are not useful for routine diagnosis but rather for research purpose. Another form of chemical profiling analysis is the culture and sensitivity assays, which involve response to chemical drug treatment. This is not a more classical routine diagnosis method but rather applicable in a situation where a pathogen's response to drug treatment is being investigated.

2.7 Entomological identification

The identification of pathogens in the arthropod vectors have been used to infer their presence in human hosts [67], wherein intermediate hosts are used as sentinels to monitor occurrence of the agents in a geographic location. Entomological survey involves catching a vector and testing with conventional molecular tool(s) to find whether they are infested with the pathogen under investigation. When vectors score positive, then deductions can be made about possible infection of humans living in that given locality. The entomological identification of agents has been applied to survey vector transmitted NTDs such as trypanosomiasis, onchocerciasis, leishmania, and dengue, in vectors including the tsetse fly, simulium fly, sandfly, and mosquitoes, respectively. The method is non-invasive for humans; hence, it reduces exposure of humans to pain associated with sample collection during disease investigation. However, the technique is only applicable to vector borne NTDs. It should also be noted that the absence of a pathogen capable of both human-to-human transmission as well as vector-to-human transmissions in a surveyed vector(s) may falsely show its absence of the in a human population if there are asymptomatic human carriers in that geographical region. Besides, where there are no vectors, it is impossible to declare absence of such infection, without conducting thorough screening of potential human reservoir. To alleviate the situation, rapid screening of potential human reservoir should be implemented concurrently. Another variant of the entomological disease investigation is performed in a confined setting where vectors are fed on a disease suspect(s), which normally present with low pathogen density with the hope of amplifying it to a detectable level in the fed vector. This method is like the isolation of pathogen by culturing techniques already reviewed in Section 2.4. Among other limitations, this method is costly considering that well-equipped infrastructure is required for maintaining vector colony for such purpose. The test result is not instant. Also, sterile vectors are fed on animal hosts, not humans, meaning that the method can only monitor vector transmitted zoonotic NTDs with known and easily accessible animal host.

2.8 Clinical manifestation

The first-line of disease investigation, in principle, is based on the detection and interpretation of symptoms to arrive at (tentative) diagnoses prior to involvement of other disease investigation methods. It is sufficed to say that clinicians in the primary healthcare often rely on disease symptoms to arrive at a diagnosis. Successful application of clinical signs to arrive at a precise diagnosis requires experience, and only works well for those diseases with cardinal signs. It should also be noted that disease detection based on symptom is usually conducted in the late stages of infection when severe damage has already occurred, making it impossible to achieve timely case management. Also, it cannot detect organisms involved in mixed infections, and latent infections often escape detection. Additionally, diseases presenting with similar signs are often impossible to discriminate. For this reason, except for a few diseases, diagnosis of NDTs based on clinical is often unreliable. Nevertheless, with all its imperfections, reliance on clinical signs is solely employed by the primary healthcare workers to diagnose tungiasis, scabies, rabies, and dracunculiasis.

3. Rapid diagnostic tests for neglected tropical diseases

Rapid diagnostic tests are characterized by their ability to give instant test result within a time span of 5 minutes to 2 hours. Such tests are essentially intended for a preliminary screening for example in resource-limited countries, where there is no easy access to healthcare [68]. Exceptionally, like during COVID-19 pandemic, they have even been used on a large scale in resource-rich countries, when the healthcare system risks of being overrun by a massive disease outbreak situation. The RDTs should meet ASSURED criteria. The commercial RDTs formats for diagnosis tests for NTDs are lateral flow immunochromatographic assays (LFIAs), agglutination-based assays, dot immunogold filtration assays (DIGFA) and LAMP. While the first three are immunoassay-based tests, and the fourth belongs is a molecular-based test. Nonetheless, many other formats of tests exist, both for the NTDs and other groups of diseases. Of recent there are also multiplex RDTs capable of detecting more than single infectious agent.

Due to the effort invested in the development of novel treatments as well as novel diagnostic tests, ten countries have eliminated at least one RDT, resulting in 500 million fewer people needing to be treated than in 2010 [69]. While progress toward the development of RTDs has been made, few tests have reached the stage of commercialization. To-date, buruli ulcer, dracunculiasis, FBT, leprosy, scabies, schistosomiasis, STH, taeniasis, cysticercosis, snakebite envenoming, and yaws still do not have reliable commercial RDTs. Although new RDTs are being developed in direct collaboration with industry [70], there remains a clear lack of interest and funding for RDTs development. Generally, less than 5% of all funding available for NTD research and development is earmarked for diagnostic development projects [69].

3.1 Formats of rapid diagnostic tests for neglected tropical diseases

Despite the limited funding available for the improvement of NTD diagnostics, the WHO's 2021–2030 road map to prevent, control, eliminate, or eradicate all 20 NTDs is enabling the development of new RDTs. At present, two formats of commercial RDTs exist; the immunoassay-based tests, and NAAT-based tests. Besides, there are hybrid tests having both immunoassay and NAAT features undergoing development [71].

3.1.1 Immunoassay-based tests

Agglutination-based tests, belonging to the immunoassay-based tests, have played a key role in the surveillance and control of leishmania and HAT in the field. Two commercial kits are commercially available through the Institute of Tropical Medicine Antwerp (Belgium) and the Academic Medical Centre Amsterdam (Netherlands) are the Card Agglutination Test for Trypanosomiasis (CATT) [72] and the Direct Agglutination Test (DAT) for leishmaniasis [73], respectively. CATT is a standard initial screening and diagnostic test for *T. brucei gambiense* HAT in the field [74, 75]. It is commercialized as a small paper sheet, for detection of parasite-induced host Abs in blood, plasma, or serum [72]. To perform the test, a sample is dispensed into the test paper, where the *T. b. gambiense* LiTat 1.3 and LiTat 1.5 VSG Ags are lyophilized attached to latex beads (**Figure 1**). When Abs recognizing these Ags are present in the test sample, they bind to multiple Ags resulting in visible agglutination [74, 76]. Similarly, DAT also detects the presence of Abs through agglutination; however, the commercial format differs. DAT is performed on 96-well plates with tip-ended wells, in which freeze-dried anti-human Abs are placed. The blood, plasma or serum sample is then applied. Right after, stained parasites are added. If Abs are present in the sample, layers of immune complex involving anti-human Ab, human anti-leishmania Ab and the leishmania Ag is formed, generating a homogenous color in the well surface [77]. In a negative test, the parasites will sink to the bottom of the wells, generating a distinct blue dot [77]. Despite their huge contribution toward the control of HAT and Leishmaniasis, CATT and DAT tests have some common drawbacks, which makes them less ideal for continued use in the field [73, 78]. Firstly, there is a problem of production robustness, resulting in the tests being mainly manufactured at research institutes. This limits the total available supplies, and requiring a cold chain to avoid spoilage [73, 75, 78]. Furthermore, both tests are not equipment free, and require electricity as well as well-trained technicians [73, 79]. In addition, the DAT has a relatively high price per test (costing about €8), and is time-consuming, requiring an incubation time of about 18 hours [73, 80]. Regarding the intrinsic properties of these tests, the sensitivity and specificity values are respectively 87–98% and 98% for

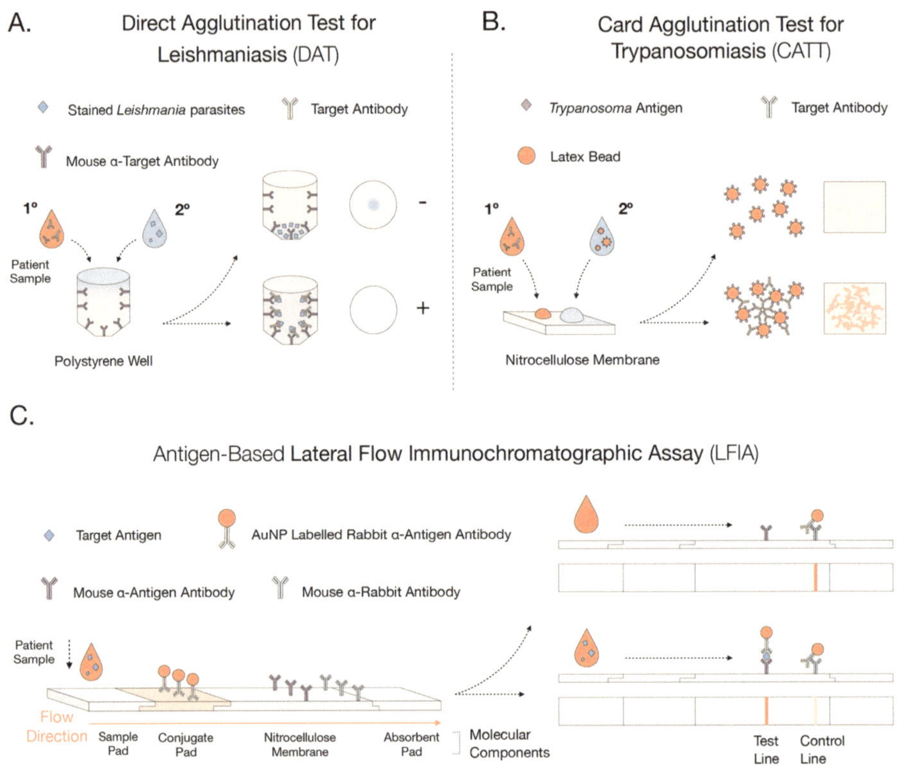

Figure 1.
Overview of the format and operating mechanism of the main commercially available immunoassay-based RDTs for the diagnosis of NTDs. A: Direct agglutination test for leishmaniasis (DAT), in which the patient sample is displayed in a polystyrene well, containing specific Abs against the target antibody. Then, stained leishmania parasites are added. In case of the presence of the target Abs, a sandwich will be formed between the capturing Abs and the stained parasites, resulting in a cloudy coloration of the well. Otherwise, a negative result will imply the parasites to sink into the well and form a clear dot. B: Card agglutination test for trypanosomiasis (CATT), in which the patient samples, and a solution with latex beads labeled with Trypanosoma antigens are displayed in a nitrocellulose membrane. In case of the presence of the target Abs, an agglutination phenomenon will be formed between the target Abs and the bead with the Ags. Otherwise, a negative result will imply the beads to be dispersed along the membrane without agglutination, resulting in a cloudy coloration of the paper. C: Antigen-based lateral flow immunochromatographic assay (LFIA), in which the patient sample is displayed in a nitrocellulose membrane, containing detecting AuNP labeled antibodies against the Ag, capturing Abs against the Ag and Abs against the detecting Abs. The sample will flow by capillary forces through the strip where, in case of the presence of the target Abs, a sandwich will be formed between the capturing and labeled detecting Abs, resulting in colored lines on the test and control lines. Otherwise, a negative result will imply the formation of a single-colored line at the control line.

CAAT, and 93–97% and 94–99% for DAT (**Table 2**). However, these values are clearly susceptible to factors such as low Ab titers, the presence of Abs from past infections, the cross-reactivity between different parasite species, or the hook effect where an excess of Abs impedes agglutination [115]. Given the low prevalence of both diseases, even a small change in specificity would result in a drastic drop in Positive Predictive Value (PPV) [2, 116]. In view of the afore-mentioned, CATT and DAT assays do not meet the ASSURED criteria, nor the recently implemented Real-time connectivity (R), and Ease (E) of specimen collection and environmental friendliness (RE) ASSURED criteria for POC diagnostic testing [117].

Point of Care applicability of RDTs has clearly been improved by the development of LFIAs for NTDs. This test format is commercially available for HAT [72], chagas

Rapid diagnostic test	Manufacturer	Target biomarker	Sensitivity (%)	Specificity (%)	Reference
		Immunoassay-based			
Card agglutination test for trypanosomiasis	ITM, Belgium	Ab α-*T. b. gambiense* Ag	87–98	98	[74]
Direct agglutination test leishmaniasis	ITM, Belgium and AMC, Netherlands	Ab α-*Labrus donovani* Ag	93–97	94–99	[73]
HAT Sero-K-SeT	Coris BioConcept, Gembloux, Belgium	Ab α-*T. b. gambiense* Ag	98–100	97–98	[72]
SD BIOLINE HAT	Abbott Laboratories, USA	Ab α-*T. b. gambiense* LiTat 1.3 and LiTat 1.5 VSG Ag	89	95	[72]
SD BIOLINE HAT 2.0	Abbott Laboratories, USA	IgG, IgM, IgA Ab α-*T. b. gambiense* VSG Ag	84–97.5	91–96.5	[72]
Bioline™ CHAGAS Ab	Abbott Laboratories, USA	Ab α-*T. cruzi* Ag	99.3	100	[81]
Chagas Detect™ Plus Rapid Test	INBIOS S.A.S., Colombia	Ab α-*T. cruzi* Ag	> 95	> 95	[82]
Trypanosoma Detect™ Rapid Test	INBIOS S.A.S., Colombia	Ab α-*T. cruzi* Ag	—	—	[83]
Chagas Antibody Test	Fortress Diagnostics, UK	Ab α-*T. cruzi* Ag	—	—	[84]
Chagas STAT-PAK assay	Chembio Diagnostics, USA	Ab α-*T. cruzi* B13, 1F8, H49/JL7 Ag	99.8	100	[85]
Bioline™ ONCHOCERCIASIS IgG4	Abbott Laboratories, USA	IgG4 Ab α-O. volvulus Ov16 Ag	81.1–85.3	99	[86]
Bioline™ CHLAMYDIA ANTIGEN TEST	Abbott Laboratories, USA	*C. trachomatis* Ag	93.1	98.8	[3]
Chlamydia Test	Fortress Diagnostics, UK	—	—	—	[87]
Chlamydia Test	Cypress Diagnostics, Belgium	—	—	—	[88]
Bioline™ DENGUE DUO	Abbott Laboratories, USA	IgG/IgM Ab α-Dengue virus and NS1 Ag	92.4–94.2	96.4–98.4	[3]
Dengue Fever IgG/IgM Antibody Test	Fortress Diagnostics, UK	IgG/ IgM Ab α-Dengue virus NS1 Ag	—	—	[89]

Rapid diagnostic test	Manufacturer	Target biomarker	Sensitivity (%)	Specificity (%)	Reference
Dengue NS1 Rapid Antigen Test	Cypress Diagnostics, Belgium	Dengue virus NS1 Ag	97.9	99	[90]
Chikungunya IgM Combo Rapid Test CE	CTK Biotech, USA	IgM Ab α-Chikungunya virus Ag	90.4	98	[91]
SD BIOLINE Chikungunya IgM	Abbott Laboratories, USA	IgM Ab α-Chikungunya virus Ag	97.1	98.9	[92]
Bioline™ LYMPHATIC FILARIASIS IgG4	Abbott Laboratories, USA	IgG4 Ab α-*W. bancrofti Wb123 Ag*	93.3–98.3	98.8–95.6	[3]
Alere™ Filariasis Test Strip	Abbott Laboratories, USA	Ab α-Wuchereria Ag	—	—	[93]
Lymphatic Filariasis rapid test kit - Brugia rapid test	Reszon Diagnostics, Malaysia	IgG4 Ab α-*B. malayi* and *B. timori* Ag	92–100	97–100	[94]
Leishmania IGG/ IGM Test	Atlas-link Biotech, China	IgG/IgM Ab α-*L. donovani* Ag	—	—	[95]
IT LEISH Individual Rapid Test	Bio-Rad, USA	Ab α-*L. donovani* rK39 Ag	86.9	82.2	[96]
Chembio Dual Path Platform rK28	Chembio Diagnostics, USA	Ab α-*L. donovani* rK28 Ag	92.3–95.9	92.5–100	[97]
Kalazar Detect™ Rapid Test for Visceral Leishmaniasis	INBIOS S.A.S., Colombia	Ab α-*L. donovani* rK39 Ag	69.2–88.7	97.4–100	[97–99]
CL Detect™ Rapid Test for Cutaneous Leishmaniasis	INBIOS S.A.S., Colombia	*Leishmania* spp. peroxidoxin Ag	96–100	84	[100]
OnSite® Leishmania Ab Rapid Test	CTK Biotech, USA	IgG/IgM Ab α-*L. donovani* rK28 Ag	92–100	98.4–100	[101]
RapiDip™ InstaTest	CTK Biotech, USA	IgG/IgM Ab α-L. donovani rK39 Ag	97–100	88–96	[102]
VIRAPID® HYDATIDOSIS	Vircell S.L., Spain	Ab α-*E. granulosus* 5/B Ag	74–94.7	96–99.5	[103, 104]
ADAMU-CE	ICST, Japan	Ab α-E. AgsEm18 Ag	57–95.8	100	[105]
Hydatidosis Rapid Test	Creative Diagnostics, USA	Abs α-*E. granulosus* Ag	—	—	[106]
Echinococcus (Echi) IgG Rapid Test	Meridian Healthcare, Italy	IgG Ab α-Echinococcus EgP164, EgP43 and EgP24 Ag	70	90	[107]
Vet-o-test Rabies Ag	BioGen Technologies, Germany	Rabies virus Ag	50–87	100	[108]

Rapid diagnostic test	Manufacturer	Target biomarker	Sensitivity (%)	Specificity (%)	Reference
Anigen Rapid Rabies Ag Test kit	Bionote, Korea	Rabies virus Ag	63.3–100	93.3–100	[109]
Quicking Pet Rapid Test	Quicking Biotech, China	Rabies virus Ag	52–57.1	100	[108]
Rapid Rabies Ag Test Kit	Creative Diagnostics, USA	Rabies virus Ag	75.6–83.3	100	[108]
Rabies Virus Ag Rapid test	Green Spring, China	Rabies virus Ag	66–83.3	100	[108]
Rabies Virus Antigen Rapid Test Kit	Abbexa Ltd., Uk	Rabies virus Ag	—	—	[110]
quickVET Rabies Antigen Rapid test	Ubio, India	Rabies virus Ag	50–52.6	100	[108]
Schisto POC-CCA®	Ict diagnostics, South Africa	IgG/IgM Ab α-*S. mansoni, S. haematobium* and *S. japonicum* Ag	70–100	—	[111]
Echinococcus DIGFA	Unibiotest, China	Ab α-*E. granulosus* EgCF, AgB and EgP Ags, and *E. multilocularis* Em2 Ag	80.7–92.9	90.3–93.4	[103, 112]
		NAAT-based			
Loopamp *T. brucei* Detection Kit	Eiken Chemical, Japan	DNA	75–90	95–100	[113]
Loopamp Leishmania Detection Kit	Eiken Chemical, Japan	DNA	85–100	100	[114]

Table 2.
A sample of commercially available rapid diagnostic tests being used for diagnosis of the neglected tropical diseases.

disease [81–85], onchocerciasis [86], Trachoma [3, 87, 88], Dengue [3, 89, 90], Chikungunya [91, 92], lymphatic filariasis [3, 93, 94], leishmaniasis [95–102], Echinococcosis [103–107], rabies [108–110], and schistosomiasis [111] (**Table 2**). These tests are based on the detection of target analytes contained in a liquid sample (i.e., body fluids such as serum, plasma, or whole blood). The analytes are displaced through capillary forces along a paper (nitrocellulose) strip, where molecules that detect the presence of the analytes are attached [118]. According to the target analyte, there are two types of LFIAs in existence: Ab-based (detecting Abs) and Ag-based (detecting Ags). LFIAs detecting Abs, upon a positive sample, will result in a sandwich formation between an Ag, adsorbed to the membrane, the target Ab, and a labeled-detection Ab. Despite the high sensitivity values usually achieved, specificity is usually limited, particularly due to the non-specific binding of non-targeted Abs with the Ags (especially when these are native antigens coming from a lysate) [119, 120]. Indeed, these tests are also inefficient when it comes to differentiating between current or past infections, as well as when performing post-treatment follow-ups [121]. In contrast, LFIAs detecting Ags, upon a positive sample, will result in a sandwich formation between the Ab, adsorbed to the membrane, the target Ag, and a labeled-detection Ab. This type of test is, in contrast to Ab-tests, able to differentiate between past and current infections, and can also be used as a test-of-cure, offering drastic improvements in the diagnosis performance of LFIAs. Moreover, their specificity values are normally much better than Ab-based tests; therefore, showing also better PPV. However, they generally have a lower sensitivity, which greatly depends on the amount of Ags in the sample [5]. This situation occurs when: (i) Ag concentration is lower than the test's analytical sensitivity or LOD (e.g., due to the masking effect produced by host anti-Ag Abs) [122]; or (ii) Ag concentration is higher than the test's concentration of detecting Abs (referred to as post-zone phenomenon of the Hook effect) [123]. Finally, it should be noted that in any LFIA, regardless of type, it is imperative to improve the method of sample extraction to make it minimally or non-invasive, thus further enhancing its applicability in the POC.

The last commercially available immunoassay-based test for RDTs (Echinococcosis) is DIGFA [103, 112]. It has a similar format to the Ab-based LFIA. However, the sandwich between the antigens on the membrane, the antibodies in the sample and the detection antibody occurs in a much similar way to an ELISA, where each reagent is added in steps, with washings in-between [112]. Although it is a test that provides a rapid result with high sensitivity and specificity values, its drawbacks remain the same as those of all the Ab-based tests mentioned above.

3.1.2 Nucleic acid-based tests

As a solution to further improve the intrinsic properties of agglutination tests, LFIA, and DIGFA (particularly for very low prevalence scenarios), the LAMP, belonging to molecular-based tests, can be used. Currently, there are commercially available LAMP assays for HAT [113], and for leishmaniasis [114]. This is a similar technique to PCR, however, enhanced for POC implementation due to the isothermal nature of the reaction (i.e., single constant temperature at around 58–65°C), only requiring a simple, low-cost heat source (e.g., a portable heat block or a water bath) [124]. Moreover, the reaction requires only 30–60 minutes to obtain a visible signal, halving that of a conventional PCR, generally without leading to non-specific amplifications [125]. Unlike PCR, LAMP amplification employs four specific primers, which can be extended to 6 by adding 2 loop primers, further reducing the reaction time [126]. In addition, it allows DNA amplification in clinical specimens (e.g., whole blood) without inhibition of their enzymes [125, 127]. LAMP readout is possible by fully quantitative techniques such as reaction tube turbidity due to magnesium pyrophosphate precipitate or color variations with pH-sensitive dyes, or by more qualitative and user-friendly methods such as LFIAs [126, 128–130]. Despite these features, LAMP reactions still have drawbacks. For instance, since it is a very sensitive technique, it is susceptible to even slight sample contaminations [127].

4. Research and development of rapid antigen tests for neglected tropical diseases

4.1 Translation of conventional immunoassays to rapid antigen tests

Conventional tests for NTDs will not be relegated completely from the disease investigation agendas, given that it is nearly impossible to develop an ideal diagnostic for each of the NTDs. Indeed, new diagnostic technologies shall only complement the existing classical assays. The current focus, therefore, should majorly aim at addressing the key limitations of the conventional tests. As such, contemporary rapid antigen detecting technologies should mainly address pitfalls bedeviling classical tests including costs, speed, portability, sensitivity, specificity, and ease of result interpretation. In recent years, conventional immunoassays have been modified to alter and/or reduce the numbers of steps, reagents, and equipment. This reduction has ultimately reduced costs, time, and risk of error often associated with multiple steps, and use of multiple reagents and equipment. Where multiple steps are involved, there are high chances of the target analyte leaching out at every step of the assays, consequently reducing the sensitivity. Non-standardized steps may also lead to high background readings, especially in ELISA when washing steps are performed sub-optimally due to time constraint. Hence, current designs of rapid Ag test are meant to minimize the factors affecting classical Ag detection test formats. Indeed, new rapid Ag tests do not require sample processing steps, use low sample volumes and some are even based on non-invasively sample collection, like saliva usage. There are also efforts being undertaken to introduce methodological modification that improve the sensitivity of RDTs. One example of this is the improvement of sensitivity of rapid Ag tests, by combining monoclonal Ag capturing antibodies with and detecting Nb reagents. Here, access and development of high affinity Nbs to a specific target antigen is important. Hence, utmost care should be exercised when screening Nb libraries, to ensure that only potent Nb molecule are selected. The most crucial activity at screening stage is to validate selected Nb molecules for interaction with their target (s) including binding affinity [131]; and, to ensure that there is no cross-reactivity with non-target antigens [4]. Authoritative protocols on Nb generation can be found elsewhere [132].

4.2 Re-designing rapid antigen diagnostic test to enhance capability using nanobodies, nanomaterials, and other technologies

Since 2003, RDTs for use in the POC had to follow the WHO-designated ASSURED criteria. However, in 2019 this term was modified to REASSURED [117]. To meet the new criteria, many improvements were introduced. Collectively, we have biosensors LFIAs, which are devices that detect the presence of an analyte present in a sample by means of a biological capture sensor (e.g., an Ab or Ag), a signal transducer (e.g., a chemically labeled-Ab), and a signal detector (e.g., absorbance or fluorescence detector) [133]. When improving, for example, the current LFIAs available for the detection of NTDs, further optimization and enhancement can be made to each of the different parts constituting the biosensor. In the following sections, some of the improvements that are undergoing investigation for future enhancement of the RDTs are discussed.

4.2.1 Nanobodies

Conventional *Gamma* (γ) immunoglobulin (IgG), have two heavy (H) and two light (L) chain polypeptides, inter-linked by inter-chain disulfide bonds [134]. Each of these chains consists of a constant domain (CH1, CH2, and CH3 for the heavy chain; and CL for the light chain), and a variable domain (VH for the heavy chain, and VL for the light chain) [135]. Generally, proteolytic cleavage of immunoglobulins (Igs) by papain and pepsin yields three and two distinct functional fragments, respectively.

Products originating from digestion of Igs by papain are two fragment antigen binding (Fab) regions, which contain both complete L chains and the CH1 and VH of the H chains; and single fragment crystallizable (Fc). On the other hand, pepsin digestion of Igs products is one F(ab')2 and may small pieces of the Fc fragment, the largest designated pFc' fragment. The Fab fragments are responsible for the binding to the target Ags by their three hyper-variable regions (CDRs), located in the VH and VL domains [136]. The Fc region (whose name refers to its easy crystallization properties), which contains paired CH2 and CH3 domains of the heavy chains is responsible for the interaction with effector molecules and cells [137].

Overall, the use of Abs as detection molecules for the development of RDTs is widely known. However, the Ab technology still has certain limitations, which have led to the exploration of novel alternatives. As it was already introduced in Section 1, the Camelidae family including *C. dromedarius*, *C. bactrianus*, *Lama glama*, *Lama guanicoe*, *Vicugna pacos*, and *V. vicugna* possess 'heavy chain-only' IgGs (HCAbs) besides convention antibodies. The cloned and expressed variable region of such HCAb is referred to as a VHH, or 'nanobody' (Nb—due to its nanometer size) [135, 138]. Nbs possess certain desirable characteristics, preferred for many applications, including the development of RDTs [5, 139]. One of these characteristics consists of their small size, being ten times smaller (~15 kDa) than conventional Abs (~150 kDa), and around 3 time smaller than a Fab (~50 kDa) [137, 140]. Despite their small size, Nbs possess the full antigen-binding potential of the parent HCAb molecule and are thereby considered to be the smallest naturally occurring intact Fabs [141]. The specific detection of antigen epitopes by Nbs primarily relies on the use of their CDR3, which unlike human Abs (with average 12 amino acids long) is commonly extended (with average 18 amino acids long) [141]. As a result, Nbs have a protruding loop that can bind to buried epitopes in the cavities (e.g., hydrophobic pockets in catalytic sites), generally inaccessible by regular Abs [142, 143]. The unique epitope preference by the Nbs and Abs partly addresses the low sensitivity problem of the Ag-based tests attributed to the immune complex masking effects [141].

Another major feature of Nbs lies in their lack of a VL region. This has resulted in natural substitutions among several of their residues, leading to a general decrease in hydrophobicity (excluding most lama spp. VHH). These amino acid substitutions are (VH-VHH): Leu12Ser, Val42Phe/Tyr, Gly49Glu, Leu50Arg/Cys, and Trp52Gly [144]. As a result, Nbs are generally: (i) more stable (resistant to high temperature-pH variations, proteolytic degradation, exposure to chemical denaturants, etc., without negatively affecting the Ag binding capacity); (ii) undergo more efficient refolding after a denaturing process, and (iii) are more soluble than conventional Abs [141]. In addition, Nbs are also easier to produce than Abs, lacking post-translational modifications and achieving higher production yields in diverse organisms (e.g., *E. coli*, *Saccharomyces cerevisiae* or *Pichia pastoris*) [141, 144, 145].

Together, these properties above have made the use of Nbs as an alternative reagent for Abs possible in many applications, including therapeutics. Examples of such applications that have been commercialized are Caplacizumab, for Thrombotic thrombocytopenic purpura [146], and Ozoralizumab, for Rheumatoid arthritis [147]. Nbs for diagnostics include NeutrobodyPlex (under development), for COVID-19 (SARS-CoV-2) [148], and Nano-IC, for acute gastroenteritis (Human Norovirus) [9]. In this regard, nanobodies have proved to be a great advantage, broadening the range of potential targets, and improving the intrinsic properties of previous tests (e.g., sensitivity of Ag-based tests). In line with diagnostics, Nb technology is being explored as a tool for development of tests for diseases caused by the Trypanosoma sp. There is ongoing development of antigen detection diagnostics including a specific Nb-based ELISA and LFIA for *T. congolense* infections [4, 5], a specific Nb-based ELISA for *T. evansi*, *T. brucei*, and *T. equiperdum* infections [149], and a Nb-based ELISA for *T. evansi*, *T. brucei*, *T. congolense*, *T. vivax* infections [150]. In addition, a Nb-based ELISA has been developed for the diagnosis of *Plasmodium falciparum* infections [151], as well as for the diagnosis of *Taenia solium* infections [152]. The relevance of Nb detection technology for the generation of new and improved RDTs for NTDs is therefore clear.

4.2.2 Nanomaterials

Since their development, LFIAs have been the preferred format for RDTs at the POC and this has been clearly confirmed after their extended use during COVID-19 pandemic. While the basic components of LFIAs technology were developed many decades ago, the integration of new nanomaterials has further improved the intrinsic properties of these tests in the recent years. These include sensitivity, specificity, PPV) and NPV. Even so, sensitivity remains the characteristic where most effort has been put into improvement, as it is often impaired in LFIAs due to low analyte concentrations in the sample [153]. Nanomaterial-based sensitivity enhancements mainly focus on: (i) improving signal transducers, or (ii) improving signal amplification.

The most used signal transducers are gold nanoparticles (AuNPs) and dyed beads, usually linked to capture antibodies. They present a low molar absorptivity, which implies that in cases of low target analyte concentration, insufficient accumulation of these nanoparticles will occur to generate a measurable optical signal [154]. Consequently, the LFIAs' sensitivity is significantly diminished. In response, research into new signal transducers has led to improvements in the LOD of the test, thereby improving sensitivity. Some of these new nanomaterials base their readability, in the same way as AuNPs or dyed beads, on their absorptivity. However, they generally have higher absorbances and more available binding sites for the detecting Abs, thus generating an overall greater contrast with the nitrocellulose strip, thereby improving the assay readout. Among these new materials are carbon nanoparticles and multi-walled carbon nanotubes, which have respectively yielded 3.8 times lower LODs and 10 times lower LODs compared to standard AuNP-based LFIAs [155, 156]. Other signal transducer improvements are based on the use of materials that allow a fluorescence-based readout. Thus, switching from a bright background readout (absorbance) to a dark background, enabling detection of minimum light levels [154]. Among these new materials are Quantum dots (QDs) and fluorescent nanodiamonds, which have respectively yielded a 78 times higher sensitivity and 105 times higher sensitivity compared to standard AuNP-based LFIAs [157, 158]. However, it is vital for fluorescence-based readout to choose a suitable strip material (e.g., nitrocellulose, or glass). If the strip materials produce auto-fluorescence at the same/near wavelength as the chosen fluorophore molecule, this will result in an intrinsic background that will impair the test performance [159].

Despite the remarkable improvements in the sensitivity of fluorescence-based readout signal transducers, the need for extra instrumentation to perform the test poses a clear drawback to its applicability in the POC [154]. A direct example of the use of these new signal transducers for the diagnosis of NTDs can be found in Dutta et al., where a test for the detection of Dengue Virus DNA with a femtomolar LOD is described [160].

Above-mentioned signal transducers are widely used in LFIAs. However, other types of diagnostic tests such as electroanalytical diagnostic methods are also under research. These typically use transistors acting as signal transducers, upon which a biological capture sensor is functionalized. When a certain voltage is applied across the transistor, if the target analyte binds to the sensor, an electrical signal is produced. This can be directly monitored by an electronic device connected to the detector. There are different approaches for such tests, which can use Abs (or even Nbs) as biological sensors, or even enzymes (e.g., Cas9) [161, 162]. Generally, these tests possess a sensitivity directly comparable to that of NAAT-based tests. However, these tests are still under development, and require further improvements to be able to directly compete with LFIAs, which are more intuitive, cost-effective, and are built with environmentally friendly materials. A few examples of this technology can be found for NTDs, for example, targeting Dengue infections [163, 164].

The enhancement of signal amplification also allows further LFIA sensitivity improvement. Several methods are available, but the most common approach is the AuNP enlargement. This involves the enhancement of the contrast produced between the AuNP color and the strip background color by bonding AuNPs to other molecules, for example silver (Ag), or platinum (Pt) metals. In this context, Ag staining occurs when this metal is released from nanofibers (contained in the strip itself) and reduced around the AuNPs. This results in 10 times more sensitivity than using AuNPs alone, and without compromising the POC properties of the LFIA [165]. The use of Pt as a sensitivity enhancement works slightly different. This metal is directly coated to AuNPs when manufacturing the strip, and has a unique feature that makes it ideal for this type of use: it has horseradish peroxidase-like catalytic activity, i.e., in the presence of 3,3′,5,5′-Tetramethylbenzidine substrate, it leads to its oxidation and generating a bluish color. This allows for up to a 100-fold increase in sensitivity, as compared to when using AuNPs alone [166].

4.2.3 Other new molecular technologies

Alternative approaches being used to improve RDTs include the use of biological capture sensors (e.g., aptamers), or the use of new strategies based on signal amplification (e.g., CRISPR-Cas). Notwithstanding the widespread use of biological capture sensors such as Abs/Nbs or Ags, it is also possible to use aptamers, nucleic acid sequences (i.e., short-stranded DNA or RNA) or peptides, which are capable of specifically binding to analytes of interest thanks to their three-dimensional conformations. Their selection and performance are comparable to that of common Abs, obtaining a robust and specific binding [167]. In addition, the low molecular weight, chemical composition, and selection process make these sensors a reliable tool with low non-specific interactions, whether with proteins, nucleic acids, or other targets [154]. Furthermore, they are more stable at high temperature conditions than Abs, thus being ideal for use in a POC setting [168, 169]. However, these tests are not yet fully optimized, meaning they are not yet cost-effective for commercialization [170].

The use of the CRISPR-Cas recognition systems as a signal amplification strategy for RDTS has been reported to increase both sensitivity and specificity, a critical requirement where disease prevalence is low, such as in HAT or leishmaniasis [116, 154]. The technology is based on the use of the RNA-guided DNA endonuclease Cas, which can be programmed to target a specific DNA/RNA sequence using a synthetic guide-RNA fragment.

Some Cas family members (e.g., Cas12, Cas13, and Cas14) remain active after cleavage of target DNAs, and execute an additional non-specific, collateral, or trans-cleavage activity [171]. By adding to the test sample ssDNA/RNA molecular probes containing a reporter, in case of the presence of the target DNA/RNA, Cas protein will start with this non-specific cleavage of surrounding probes, releasing the reporter molecules, easily detected with a LFIA [172]. In addition, this method can be coupled to RDTs such as LAMP, resulting in considerable improvements in sensitivity and specificity [173], at a reduced price per test (as low as $0.61 USD) [174, 175]. Although not yet commercially available, mainly due to the lack of pre-amplification optimization prior to the use of this technology, there are already examples of reported use for diagnosis of NTDs such as for HAT [71], Zika and Dengue [157].

5. Conclusion

There is hope of overcoming the burdens of NTDs and other diseases, currently contributing to the development challenges facing low-income countries. Effective ways to contain these diseases are early detection, case management, periodic surveillance, and implementation of preventive measures including regular sensitization of the masses through community awareness campaigns. In the recent past the WHO has drawn attention for the need to combat the scourge of NTDs. Although there are positive gains following the ongoing WHO campaign, it is important to realize that some of the NTDs cannot be diagnose effectively due to the lack of proper diagnostics. Therefore, new technologies should be developed to improve or complement the existing diagnostic platforms. Preferably, these new diagnostic inventions should be REASSURED. With all its desirable attributes, Nb technology is a new technology not yet maximally explored in the fields of NTD diagnostics. Except for prototypes—developed for only a few NTDs including cysticercosis and animal trypanosomiasis—there are no commercial Nb-based RDTs for NTDs. There is need to deeply investigate the potentials of Nbs for diagnosis of NTDs currently left unattended. As a first step to this approach, researchers should dedicate efforts to finding suitable biomarker(s) for each of the NTDs where applicable. Thereafter, Nbs should be generated against each of these target profiles followed by assay development and proper validation. For this to succeed, there is urgent need for cooperation among relevant stakeholders including the WHO, development agencies including non-governmental organizations, commercial companies, industries, research scientists, clinicians, policy makers, economists, research and/or education institutions, as well as community leaders.

A. Definitions of key parameters of diagnostic tests

A 2 × 2 table showing how to analyze diagnostic test parameters. The information presented in the table originated from [176].

New diagnostic test result	Reference standard true diagnosis		Total
	Positive	Negative	
Positive	*a* (True positive)	*b* (False negative)	*a* + *b*
Negative	*c* (False positive)	*d* (True negative)	c + *d*
Total	(*a* + *c*)	(*b* + *d*)	(*N*)

(i) Diagnostic Accuracy:[(a + d)/N]; (ii) Sensitivity: the test's ability to obtain a positive test when the target condition is really present, or the true positive rate [a/(a + c)]; (iii) Specificity: the test's ability to obtain a negative test when the condition is really absent, or the true negative rate [d/(b + d)]; (iv) False positive rate (1 - specificity): the probability of an incorrect positive test in those who do not have the target condition [b/(b + d)]; (v) False negative rate (1 - sensitivity): the probability of obtaining an incorrect negative test in patients who do have the target disorder [c/(a + c)]; (vi) Positive Predictive Value (PPV): the proportion of the true positive in those samples that scored positive by the test [a/(a + b)]; (vii) Negative Predictive Value (NPV): the proportion of true negative in those sample that scored negative by test [d/(c + d)]; (viii) Prevalence: the number of cases of a condition existing in each population at any one time [(a + c)/N]; (ix) Positive likelihood ratio: tell us how many times more likely a positive test will be seen in those with the disorder than in those without the disorder *[Sensitivity/1 – Specificity*]; and (x) Negative likelihood ratio: tell us how many times more likely a negative test will be seen in those with the disorder than in those without the disorder [*1 - Sensitivity/Specificity*].

Acknowledgements

This work was supported by a SB PhD fellowship of the Research Foundation – Flanders (FWO), project number 1S91223N.

Author details

Andrés Álvarez-Rodríguez[1,2], Magdalena Radwanska[3,4], Stefan Magez[1,2,3] and Steven Odongo[3,5,6]*

1 Laboratory of Cellular and Molecular Immunology, Vrije Universiteit Brussel, Brussels, Belgium

2 Department of Biomedical Biochemistry and Microbiology, Ghent University, Ghent, Belgium

3 Laboratory for Biomedical Research, Ghent University Global Campus, Incheon, South Korea

4 Department of Biomedical Molecular Biology, Ghent University, Ghent, Belgium

5 Department of Biotechnical and Diagnostic Sciences, College of Veterinary Medicine, Animal Resources and Biosecurity, Makerere University, Kampala, Uganda

6 Center for Biosecurity and Global Health, College of Veterinary Medicine, Animal Resources and Biosecurity, Makerere University, Kampala, Uganda

*Address all correspondence to: steven.odongo@ghent.ac.kr; steven.odongo@mak.ac.ug

References

[1] WHO. The Top 10 Causes of Death [Internet]. 2022. Available from: https://www.who.int/news-room/fact-sheets/detail/the-top-10-causes-of-death. [Accessed: November 28, 2022]

[2] Ntuli MM, editors. Ending the neglect to attain the Sustainable Development Goals: A Road Map for Neglected Tropical Diseases 2021–2030. World Health Organization; 2020. 196 p. ISBN: 978 92 4 001035 2. Available from: https://www.who.int/publications/i/item/9789240010352. [Accessed: December 11, 2022]

[3] Bioline. Rapid Diagnostic Test Infectious Diseases, Bioline TM Product Catalogue [Internet]. 2022. Available from: https://content.veeabb.com/1d09429b-8373-419f-8f1a-d28f9586863a/87c102d8-0a11-45f2-925f-c3ffae2d2345/87c102d8-0a11-45f2-925f-c3ffae2d2345_source__v.pdf [Accessed: November 28, 2022]

[4] Odongo S et al. An anti-proteome nanobody library approach yields a specific immunoassay for Trypanosoma congolense diagnosis targeting glycosomal aldolase. PLoS Neglected Tropical Diseases. 2016;**10**(2): e0004420. DOI: 10.1371/journal.pntd.0004420

[5] Torres JE et al. Development of a nanobody-based lateral flow assay to detect active Trypanosoma congolense infections. Scientific Reports. 2018;**8**(1):9019. DOI: 10.1038/s41598-018-26732-7

[6] Büscher P. Diagnosis of African trypanosomiasis. In: Magez S, Radwanska M, editors. Trypanosomes and Trypanosomiasis. Wien: Springer; 2014. pp. 189-216. DOI: 10.1007/978-3-7091-1556-5_8

[7] Muyldermans S et al. Camelid immunoglobulins and nanobody technology. Veterinary Immunology and Immunopathology. 2009;**128**(1–3): 178-183. DOI: 10.1016/j.vetimm.2008.10.299

[8] Hamers-Casterman C et al. Naturally occurring antibodies devoid of light chains. Nature. 1993;**363**(6428): 446-448. DOI: 10.1038/363446a0

[9] Doerflinger SY et al. Development of a nanobody-based lateral flow immunoassay for detection of human norovirus. mSphere. 2016;**1**(5):e00219-16. DOI: 10.1128/mSphere.00219-16

[10] Zhang C et al. Development of nanobody-based flow-through dot ELISA and lateral-flow immunoassay for rapid detection of 3-phenoxybenzoic acid. Analytical Methods. 2021;**13**(14): 1757-1765. DOI: 10.1039/d1ay00129a

[11] Salvador JP, Vasylieva N, Gonzalez-Garcia I, Jin M, Caster R, Siegel JB, et al. Nanobody-based lateral flow immunoassay for the rapid detection of aflatoxin B1 in almond milk. ACS Food Science & Technology. 2022;**2**(8): 1276-1282. DOI: 10.1021/acsfoodscitech.2c00118

[12] Desmyter A et al. Crystal structure of a camel single-domain VH antibody fragment in complex with lysozyme. Nature Structural Biology. 1996;**3**(9): 803-811. DOI: 10.1038/nsb0996-803

[13] De Genst E et al. Molecular basis for the preferential cleft recognition by dromedary heavy-chain antibodies. Proceedings of the National Academy of Sciences of the United States of America. 2006;**103**(12):4586-4591. DOI: 10.1073/pnas.0505379103

[14] Crowther JR. Methods in Molecular Biology: The ELISA Guidebook. 2nd ed. New York: Springer Science; 2009. p. 413. DOI: 10.1385/1592590497

[15] Mullis KB. The unusual origin of the polymerase chain reaction. Scientific American. 1990;**262**(4):56-61, 64-5. DOI: 10.1038/scientificamerican0490-56

[16] Stinear T et al. Identification and characterization of IS2404 and IS2606: Two distinct repeated sequences for detection of *Mycobacterium ulcerans* by PCR. Journal of Clinical Microbiology. 1999;**37**(4):1018-1023. DOI: 10.1128/JCM.37.4.1018-1023.1999

[17] Lanciotti RS et al. Rapid detection and typing of dengue viruses from clinical samples by using reverse transcriptase-polymerase chain reaction. Journal of Clinical Microbiology. 1992; **30**(3):545-551. DOI: 10.1128/jcm.30.3.545-551.1992

[18] Van Den Bossche D, Cnops L, Meersman K, Domingo C, Van Gompel A, Van Esbroeck M. Chikungunya virus and West Nile virus infections imported into Belgium, 2007-2012. Epidemiology and Infection. 2015;**143**(10):2227-2236. DOI: 10.1017/S0950268814000685

[19] Radwanska M et al. The serum resistance-associated gene as a diagnostic tool for the detection of Trypanosoma brucei rhodesiense. The American Journal of Tropical Medicine and Hygiene. 2002;**67**(6):684-690. DOI: 10.4269/ajtmh.2002.67.684

[20] Hijjawi N et al. Molecular diagnosis and identification of leishmania species in Jordan from saved dry samples. BioMed Research International. 2016; **2016**:6871739. DOI: 10.1155/2016/6871739

[21] Coker SM et al. Development and validation of a quantitative PCR for the detection of Guinea worm (*Dracunculus medinensis*). PLoS Neglected Tropical Diseases. 2022;**16**(10):e0010830. DOI: 10.1371/journal.pntd.0010830

[22] Rodrigues AM, de Hoog GS, de Camargo ZP. Molecular diagnosis of pathogenic Sporothrix species. PLoS Neglected Tropical Diseases. 2015;**9**(12): e0004190. DOI: 10.1371/journal.pntd.0004190

[23] Biamonte MA et al. Onchocerciasis: Target product profiles of in vitro diagnostics to support onchocerciasis elimination mapping and mass drug administration stopping decisions. PLoS Neglected Tropical Diseases. 2022;**16**(8): e0010682. DOI: 10.1371/journal.pntd.0010682

[24] Mani RS, Anand AM, Madhusudana SN. Human rabies in India: An audit from a rabies diagnostic laboratory. Tropical Medicine & International Health. 2016;**21**(4): 556-563. DOI: 10.1111/tmi.12669

[25] Ngcamphalala PI, Lamb J, Mukaratirwa S. Molecular identification of hookworm isolates from stray dogs, humans and selected wildlife from South Africa. Journal of Helminthology. 2019;**94**:e39. DOI: 10.1017/S0022149X19000130

[26] Chi KH et al. Molecular differentiation of Treponema pallidum subspecies in skin ulceration clinically suspected as yaws in Vanuatu using real-time multiplex PCR and serological methods. The American Journal of Tropical Medicine and Hygiene. 2015; **92**(1):134-138. DOI: 10.4269/ajtmh.14-0459

[27] Dinkel A et al. Detection of Echinococcus multilocularis in the

definitive host: Coprodiagnosis by PCR as an alternative to necropsy. Journal of Clinical Microbiology. 1998;**36**(7): 1871-1876. DOI: 10.1128/JCM.36.7.1871-1876.1998

[28] Cox A et al. A PCR based assay for detection and differentiation of African trypanosome species in blood. Experimental Parasitology. 2005;**111**(1):24-29. DOI: 10.1016/j.exppara.2005.03.014

[29] Delespaux V et al. PCR-RFLP using Ssu-rDNA amplification: Applicability for the diagnosis of mixed infections with different trypanosome species in cattle. Veterinary Parasitology. 2003; **117**(3):185-193. DOI: 10.1016/j.vetpar.2003.08.004

[30] Reimao JQ et al. Laboratory diagnosis of cutaneous and visceral leishmaniasis: Current and future methods. Microorganisms. 2020;**8**(11): 1632. DOI: 10.3390/microorganisms 8111632

[31] Thanomsub BW et al. Differential diagnosis of human lymphatic filariasis using PCR-RFLP. Molecular and Cellular Probes. 2000;**14**(1):41-46. DOI: 10.1006/mcpr.1999.0283

[32] Mulinge E et al. Molecular identification of zoonotic hookworms in dogs from four counties of Kenya. Journal of Helminthology. 2019;**94**:e43. DOI: 10.1017/S0022149X1900018X

[33] Fyfe JA et al. Development and application of two multiplex real-time PCR assays for the detection of *Mycobacterium ulcerans* in clinical and environmental samples. Applied and Environmental Microbiology. 2007; **73**(15):4733-4740. DOI: 10.1128/AEM.02971-06

[34] Notomi T et al. Loop-mediated isothermal amplification of DNA. Nucleic Acids Research. 2000;**28**(12): E63. DOI: 10.1093/nar/28.12.e63

[35] Kuboki N et al. Loop-mediated isothermal amplification for detection of African trypanosomes. Journal of Clinical Microbiology. 2003;**41**(12): 5517-5524. DOI: 10.1128/JCM.41.12.5517-5524.2003

[36] Chen X et al. Nanoparticle-based lateral flow biosensor integrated with loop-mediated isothermal amplification for rapid and visual identification of chlamydia trachomatis for point-of-care use. Frontiers in Microbiology. 2022;**13**: 914620. DOI: 10.3389/fmicb.2022.914620

[37] Mabey D et al. Diagnostics for the developing world. Nature Reviews. Microbiology. 2004;**2**(3):231-240. DOI: 10.1038/nrmicro841

[38] Van Weemen BK, Schuurs AH. Immunoassay using antigen-enzyme conjugates. FEBS Letters. 1971;**15**(3): 232-236. DOI: 10.1016/0014-5793(71)80319-8

[39] Forsyth CJ et al. Recommendations for screening and diagnosis of chagas disease in the United States. The Journal of Infectious Diseases. 2022;**225**(9): 1601-1610. DOI: 10.1093/infdis/jiab513

[40] CDC. Centers for Disease Control and Prevention: Serologic Tests for Dengue Virus. 2019. Available from: https://www.cdc.gov/dengue/healthcare-providers/testing/serologic-tests.html

[41] Gottstein B et al. Serological (Em2-ELISA) and parasitological examinations of fox populations for Echinococcus multilocularis infections. Zentralblatt für Veterinärmedizin. Reihe B. 1991;**38**(3): 161-168. DOI: 10.1111/j.1439-0450.1991.tb00858.x

[42] Romero-Montoya M, Beltran-Alzate JC, Cardona-Castro N. Evaluation and monitoring of mycobacterium leprae transmission in household contacts of patients with Hansen's disease in Colombia. PLoS Neglected Tropical Diseases. 2017;**11**(1):e0005325. DOI: 10.1371/journal.pntd.0005325

[43] Shintouo CM et al. Tandem use of OvMANE1 and Ov-16 ELISA tests increases the sensitivity for the diagnosis of human onchocerciasis. Life (Basel). 2021;**11**(12). DOI: 10.3390/life11121284

[44] Hancock K, Tsang VC. Development and optimization of the FAST-ELISA for detecting antibodies to *Schistosoma mansoni*. Journal of Immunological Methods. 1986;**92**(2):167-176. DOI: 10.1016/0022-1759(86)90162-6

[45] Shalaby SI et al. Detection of coproantigens by Sandwich ELISA in rabbits experimentally infected with Fasciola gigantica. Iranian Journal of Parasitology. 2014;**9**(3):374-381

[46] Wattal S et al. Evaluation of Og4C3 antigen ELISA as a tool for detection of bancroftian filariasis under lymphatic filariasis elimination programme. The Journal of Communicable Diseases. 2007;**39**(2):75-84

[47] Wanji S et al. Further evidence of the cross-reactivity of the Binax NOW(R) filariasis ICT cards to non-Wuchereria bancrofti filariae: Experimental studies with Loa Loa and Onchocerca ochengi. Parasites & Vectors. 2016;**9**:267. DOI: 10.1186/s13071-016-1556-8

[48] Espino AM, Millan JC, Finlay CM. Detection of antibodies and circulating excretory-secretory antigens for assessing cure in patients with fascioliasis. Transactions of the Royal Society of Tropical Medicine and Hygiene. 1992;**86**(6):649. DOI: 10.1016/0035-9203(92)90174-b

[49] Stanley JT, Gunsalus RP, Lory S, Perry J.J. Microbial Life, 2nd ed. Sunderland, MA: Sinauer Associates; 2007. p. 1066. DOI: 10.1093/icb/icm096

[50] Madigan MT, Bender KS, Buckley DH, Brock TD, Sattley MW, Stahl DA. Biology of Microorganisms. 15th ed. Pearson; 2018. p. 1058. ISBN 1292235101, 9781292235103

[51] Riedel S, Morse S, Mietzner T, Miller S. Jawetz Melnick & Adelbergs Medical Microbiology. 28th ed. McGraw Hill/Medical; 2019. ISBN10: 1260012026 | ISBN13: 9781260012026

[52] Roepstorff A et al. Helminth parasites in pigs: New challenges in pig production and current research highlights. Veterinary Parasitology. 2011;**180**(1–2):72-81. DOI: 10.1016/j.vetpar.2011.05.029

[53] WHO/Expert Committee on the Control of human African trypanosomiasis editors. Control and surveillance of human African trypanosomiasis: WHO TRS N°984: Report of a meeting of the WHO Expert Committee. 2013. p. 247. ISBN: 978 92 4 120984 7. Available from: https://www.who.int/publications/i/item/WHO-TRS-984 [Accessed: January 01, 2023]

[54] Hay R et al. The diagnosis of fungal neglected tropical diseases (fungal NTDs) and the role of investigation and laboratory tests: An expert consensus report. Tropical Medicine and Infectious Disease. 2019;**4**(4):122. DOI: 10.3390/tropicalmed4040122

[55] Speich B et al. Comparative cost assessment of the Kato-Katz and FLOTAC techniques for soil-transmitted helminth diagnosis in epidemiological

surveys. Parasites & Vectors. 2010;**3**:71. DOI: 10.1186/1756-3305-3-71

[56] Dofitas BL et al. Yaws in the Philippines: First reported cases since the 1970s. Infectious Diseases of Poverty. 2020;**9**(1):1. DOI: 10.1186/s40249-019-0617-6

[57] Barthold SW, Bowen RA, Hedrick RP, Knowels DP, Lairmore MD, Parrish CR. In: Maclachlan NJ, Dubovi EJ, editors. Fenner's Veterinary Virology. 4th ed. Oxford: Elsevier Inc.; 2010. p. 507. DOI: 10.1016/C2013-0-06921-6

[58] Rodriguez Carnero P et al. Unexpected hosts: Imaging parasitic diseases. Insights Into Imaging. 2017; **8**(1):101-125. DOI: 10.1007/s13244-016-0525-2

[59] Barry SK, Schucany WG. Dracunculiasis of the breast: Radiological manifestations of a rare disease. Journal of Radiology Case Reports. 2012;**6**(11):29-33. DOI: 10.3941/jrcr.v6i11.1137

[60] Caglar YS et al. Spinal hydatid cyst disease : Challenging surgery—An institutional experience. Journal of Korean Neurosurgical Association. 2019; **62**(2):209-216. DOI: 10.3340/jkns.2017.0245

[61] Brown JD. Human fascioliasis (liver fluke disease) in Hawai'i: Case report and review of human fascioliasis acquired in the United States. Hawai'i Journal of Health & Social Welfare. 2021;**80**(9):212-217

[62] Mand S et al. Frequent detection of worm movements in onchocercal nodules by ultrasonography. Filaria Journal. 2005;**4**(1):1. DOI: 10.1186/1475-2883-4-1

[63] Garcia HH, Gonzalez AE, Gilman RH. Taenia solium cysticercosis and its impact in neurological disease. Clinical Microbiology Reviews. 2020;**33**(3): e00085-19. DOI: 10.1128/CMR.00085-19

[64] Converse PJ et al. Accelerated detection of mycolactone production and response to antibiotic treatment in a mouse model of mycobacterium ulcerans disease. PLoS Neglected Tropical Diseases. 2014;**8**(1):e2618. DOI: 10.1371/journal.pntd.0002618

[65] Van der Auwera G, Dujardin JC. Species typing in dermal leishmaniasis. Clinical Microbiology Reviews. 2015; **28**(2):265-294. DOI: 10.1128/CMR.00104-14

[66] Papadopoulos MC et al. A novel and accurate diagnostic test for human African trypanosomiasis. Lancet. 2004; **363**(9418):1358-1363. DOI: 10.1016/S0140-6736(04)16046-7

[67] Cameron MM, Ramesh A. The use of molecular xenomonitoring for surveillance of mosquito-borne diseases. Philosophical Transactions of the Royal Society of London. Series B, Biological Sciences. 1818;**2021**(376):20190816. DOI: 10.1098/rstb.2019.0816

[68] Gashaw T, Hagos B, Sisay M. Expected impacts of COVID-19: Considering resource-limited countries and vulnerable population. Frontiers in Public Health. 2021;**9**:614789. DOI: 10.3389/fpubh.2021.614789

[69] FIND. Marginalized populations. 2022. Available from: https://www.finddx.org/marginalized-populations/

[70] Wadagni A et al. Simple, rapid Mycobacterium ulcerans disease diagnosis from clinical samples by fluorescence of Mycolactone on thin

layer chromatography. PLoS Neglected Tropical Diseases. 2015;**9**(11):e0004247. DOI: 10.1371/journal.pntd.0004247

[71] Sima N et al. SHERLOCK4HAT: A CRISPR-based tool kit for diagnosis of human African trypanosomiasis. eBioMedicine. 2022;**85**:104308. DOI: 10.1016/j.ebiom.2022.104308

[72] Bottieau E, Clerinx J. Human African trypanosomiasis: Progress and stagnation. Infectious Disease Clinics of North America. 2019;**33**(1):61-77. DOI: 10.1016/j.idc.2018.10.003

[73] Kuhne V, Buscher P. The unknown nature of the antigen in the direct agglutination test for visceral leishmaniasis hampers development of serodiagnostic tests. The American Journal of Tropical Medicine and Hygiene. 2019;**100**(2):246-255. DOI: 10.4269/ajtmh.18-0740

[74] Magnus E, Vervoort T, Van Meirvenne N. A card-agglutination test with stained trypanosomes (C.A.T.T.) for the serological diagnosis of T. B. gambiense trypanosomiasis. Annales de la Société Belge de Médecine Tropicale. 1978;**58**(3):169-176

[75] Lejon V et al. The separation of trypanosomes from blood by anion exchange chromatography: From Sheila Lanham's discovery 50 years ago to a gold standard for sleeping sickness diagnosis. PLoS Neglected Tropical Diseases. 2019;**13**(2):e0007051. DOI: 10.1371/journal.pntd. 0007051

[76] Penchenier L et al. Evaluation of LATEX/*T.b.gambiense* for mass screening of *Trypanosoma brucei gambiense* sleeping sickness in Central Africa. Acta Tropica. 2003;**85**(1): 31-37. DOI: 10.1016/s0001-706x(02) 00232-2

[77] Farahmand M et al. Assessment of recombinant A2-latex agglutination test (RA2-LAT) and RA2-ELISA for detection of canine visceral leishmaniasis: A comparative field study with direct agglutination test in Northwestern Iran. Iranian Journal of Parasitology. 2018;**13**(2):172-179

[78] Hasker E et al. A new format of the CATT test for the detection of human African trypanosomiasis, designed for use in peripheral health facilities. Tropical Medicine & International Health. 2010;**15**(2):263-267. DOI: 10.1111/j.1365-3156.2009.02446.x

[79] Lumbala C et al. Prospective evaluation of a rapid diagnostic test for *Trypanosoma brucei gambiense* infection developed using recombinant antigens. PLoS Neglected Tropical Diseases. 2018; **12**(3):e0006386. DOI: 10.1371/journal. pntd.0006386

[80] Schallig HD, Canto-Cavalheiro M, da Silva ES. Evaluation of the direct agglutination test and the rK39 dipstick test for the sero-diagnosis of visceral leishmaniasis. Memórias do Instituto Oswaldo Cruz. 2002;**97**(7):1015-1018. DOI: 10.1590/s0074-027620020007 00015

[81] Abbott. Bioline™ CHAGAS Ab ANTIBODY TEST FOR TRYPANOSOMA CRUZI (CHAGAS) [Internet]. 2022. Available from: https:// chembio.com/products/chagas-stat-pak-assay-europe/ [Accessed: December 23, 2022]

[82] InBios-International. Chagas Detect™ Plus Rapid Test: FDA Cleared for In Vitro Diagnostic Use in the United States [Internet]. 2022. Available from: https://inbios.com/chagas-detecttm-plus-rapid-test-intl-fda-cleared/ [Accessed: December 03, 2022]

[83] InBios-International. Trypanosoma Detect™ Rapid Test [Internet]. 2022. Available from: https://inbios.com/trypanosoma-detecttm-rapid-test-intl/ [Accessed: December 23, 2022]

[84] Diagnostics, F. Chagas Antibody Test [Internet]. 2022. Available from: https://www.fortressdiagnostics.com/products/rapid-diagnostic-tests/chagas-antibody-test [Accessed: December 30, 2022]

[85] CHEMBIO. Chagas STAT PAK® Assay: Rapidly Detect Chagas Infection [Internet]. 2022. Available from: https://chembio.com/products/chagas-stat-pak-assay-europe/ [Accessed: December 20, 2022]

[86] Abbott. Bioline™ ONCHO/IF IGG4 Biplex: New Tools to Support Disease Elimination for Both River Blindness and Elephantiasis [Internet]. 2022. Available from: https://www.globalpointofcare.abbott/en/product-details/bioline-onchocerciasis-LF-igg4-rapid-test.html [Accessed: December 03, 2022]

[87] Fotress-Diagnostics. Chlamydia Test [Internet]. 2022. Available from: https://www.fortressdiagnostics.com/products/rapid-diagnostic-tests/chlamydia-test [Accessed: December 08, 2022]

[88] Cypress-Diagnostics. Chlamydia Ag. [Internet]. 2022. Available from: https://diagnostics.be/fr/product/322 [Accessed: December 03, 2022]

[89] Diagnostics, F. Dengue Fever [Internet]. 2022. Available from: https://www.fortressdiagnostics.com/products/rapid-diagnostic-tests/dengue-fever [Accessed: December 09, 2022]

[90] Cypress-Diagnostics. Dengue NS1 Rapid Antigen Test for Dengue Fever [Internet]. 2022. Available from: https://fgmdiagnostici.it/files/78.pdf [Accessed: December 05, 2022]

[91] CTK-Biotech. Chikungunya IgM Combo Rapid Test CE [Internet]. 2022. Available from: https://ctkbiotech.com/product/chikungunya-igm-combo-rapid-test-ce/ [Accessed: December 15, 2022]

[92] Abbott. SD BIOLINE Chikungunya IgM: One Step IgM antibodies to Chikungunya virus Test [Internet]. 2022. Available from: https://maxanim.com/content/abbott/sd-bioline/sd-bioline-chikungunya-igm.pdf [Accessed: December 15, 2022]

[93] Abbott. AlereTM Filariasis Test Strip [Internet]. 2022. Available from: https://www.cor-ntd.org/sites/default/files/content/document/FTS_v2_07JUL2016.pdf [Accessed: December 15, 2022]

[94] Reszon-Diagnostics. LYMPHATIC FILARIASIS RAPID TEST KIT BRUGIA RAPID TEST [Internet]. 2022. Available from: https://reszonics.com/products/infectious-diseases-diagnosis/lateral-flow-rapid-test/brugia-rapid-test/ [Accessed: December 15, 2022]

[95] Ease-Medtrend-Biotech. Leishmania IGG/IGM Test [Internet]. 2022. Available from: http://www.atlas-link.com/english/product_s33.html [Accessed: December 21, 2022]

[96] Bio-Rad. IT LEISH Individual Rapid Test [Internet]. 2022. Available from: https://www.bio-rad.com/sites/default/files/webroot/web/pdf/cdg/literature/16490_B-IT_LEISH-EN.pdf [Accessed: December 15, 2022]

[97] Pattabhi S et al. Design, development and evaluation of rK28-based point-of-care tests for

improving rapid diagnosis of visceral leishmaniasis. PLoS Neglected Tropical Diseases. 2010;**4**(9): e0000822. DOI: 10.1371/journal.pntd.0000822

[98] Hagos DG et al. Performance of rapid rk39 tests for the diagnosis of visceral leishmaniasis in Ethiopia: A systematic review and meta-analysis. BMC Infectious Diseases. 2021;**21**(1): 1166. DOI: 10.1186/s12879-021-06826-w

[99] InBios-International. Kalazar Detect™ Rapid Test for Visceral Leishmaniasis [Internet]. 2022. Available from: https://inbios.com/kalazar-detecttm-rapid-test-for-visceral-leishmaniasis-intl/ [Accessed: December 21, 2022]

[100] InBios-International. CL Detect™ Rapid Test for Cutaneous Leishmaniasis [Internet]. 2022. Available from: https://inbios.com/cl-detecttm-rapid-test-for-cutaneous-leishmaniasis-intl/ [Accessed: December 26, 2022]

[101] CTK-Biotech. OnSite Leishmania Ab Rapid Test—Strip (Serum/Plasma) [Internet]. 2022. Available from: https://athenesedx.com/insert/R0122S.pdf [Accessed: December 19, 2022]

[102] CTK-Biotech. Leishmania Ab Rapid Test CE [Internet]. 2022. Available from: https://ctkbiotech.com/product/leishmania-ab-rapid-test-ce/ [Accessed: December 21, 2022]

[103] Tamarozzi F et al. Comparison of the diagnostic accuracy of three rapid tests for the serodiagnosis of hepatic cystic echinococcosis in humans. PLoS Neglected Tropical Diseases. 2016;**10**(2): e0004444. DOI: 10.1371/journal.pntd.0004444

[104] Vircell-S.L. VIRAPID® HYDATIDOSIS [Internet]. 2022. Available from: https://www.vircell.com/producto/virapid-hydatidosis/ [Accessed: December 10, 2022]

[105] ICST. ADAMU-CE [Internet]. 2022. Available from: https://icst.jp/english/products/pdf/adamu_ce_en.pdf [Accessed: December 26, 2022]

[106] Creative-Diagnostics. Hydatidosis Rapid Test. 2022. Available from: https://www.creative-diagnostics.com/Hydatidosis-Test-132038-453.htm

[107] Meridian-Healthcare. Echinococcus (Echi) IgG Rapid Test [Internet]. 2022. Available from: https://www.meridianhealthcare.it/echinococco-echi-igg-rapid-test/?lang=en [Accessed: December 15, 2022]

[108] Eggerbauer E et al. Evaluation of six commercially available rapid immunochromatographic tests for the diagnosis of rabies in brain material. PLoS Neglected Tropical Diseases. 2016; **10**(6):e0004776. DOI: 10.1371/journal.pntd.0004776

[109] Lechenne M et al. Validation of a rapid rabies diagnostic tool for field surveillance in developing countries. PLoS Neglected Tropical Diseases. 2016; **10**(10):e0005010. DOI: 10.1371/journal.pntd.0005010

[110] Abbexa-Ltd. Rabies Virus Antigen Rapid Test Kit [Internet]. 2022. Available from: https://www.abbexa.com/rabies-virus-antigen-rapid-test-kit-colloidal-gold [Accessed: December 10, 2022]

[111] Ict-diagnostics, Schisto POC-CCA®: Rapid test for qualitative detection of: Bilharzia (Schistosomiasis) [Internet]. 2022. Available from: http://www.ictdiagnostics.co.za/schistosomanew.html [Accessed: December 19, 2022]

[112] Feng X et al. Dot immunogold filtration assay (DIGFA) with multiple native antigens for rapid serodiagnosis of human cystic and alveolar echinococcosis. Acta Tropica. 2010; **113**(2):114-120. DOI: 10.1016/j.acta tropica.2009.10.003

[113] Njiru ZK et al. African trypanosomiasis: Sensitive and rapid detection of the sub-genus Trypanozoon by loop-mediated isothermal amplification (LAMP) of parasite DNA. International Journal for Parasitology. 2008;**38**(5):589-599. DOI: 10.1016/j. ijpara.2007.09.006

[114] Hossain F et al. Evaluation of Loopamp leishmania detection kit and leishmania antigen ELISA for post-elimination detection and Management of Visceral Leishmaniasis in Bangladesh. Frontiers in Cellular and Infection Microbiology. 2021;**11**:670759. DOI: 10.3389/fcimb.2021.670759

[115] Gillet P et al. Assessment of the prozone effect in malaria rapid diagnostic tests. Malaria Journal. 2009;**8**: 271. DOI: 10.1186/1475-2875-8-271

[116] Alvarez-Rodriguez A et al. Recent progress in diagnosis and treatment of human African trypanosomiasis has made the elimination of this disease a realistic target by 2030. Frontiers in Medicine. 2022;**9**:1037094. DOI: 10.3389/fmed.2022.1037094

[117] Land KJ et al. REASSURED diagnostics to inform disease control strategies, strengthen health systems and improve patient outcomes. Nature Microbiology. 2019;**4**(1):46-54. DOI: 10.1038/s41564-018-0295-3

[118] Koczula KM, Gallotta A. Lateral flow assays. Essays in Biochemistry. 2016;**60**(1):111-120. DOI: 10.1042/ EBC20150012

[119] Desquesnes M et al. The analysis of the cross-reactions occurring in antibody-ELISA for the detection of trypanosomes can improve identification of the parasite species involved. Annals of Tropical Medicine and Parasitology. 2001;**95**(2):141-155. DOI: 10.1080/ 00034980120050251

[120] Lejon V et al. Performance of enzyme-linked immunosorbent assays for detection of antibodies against *T. congolense* and *T. vivax* in goats. Veterinary Parasitology. 2003;**116**(2): 87-95. DOI: 10.1016/s0304-4017(03) 00257-7

[121] Kennedy PGE. Update on human African trypanosomiasis (sleeping sickness). Journal of Neurology. 2019; **266**(9):2334-2337. DOI: 10.1007/ s00415-019-09425-7

[122] Büscher P. Diagnosis of human and animal African trypanosomiasis. In: Black SJ, Seed JR, editors. The African Trypanosomes. New York: Kluwer Academic Publishers; 2002. pp. 51-63. DOI: 10.1007/0-306-46894-8_5

[123] Ross GMS et al. Unraveling the hook effect: A comprehensive study of high antigen concentration effects in Sandwich lateral flow immunoassays. Analytical Chemistry. 2020;**92**(23): 15587-15595. DOI: 10.1021/acs. analchem.0c03740

[124] Niemz A, Ferguson TM, Boyle DS. Point-of-care nucleic acid testing for infectious diseases. Trends in Biotechnology. 2011;**29**(5):240-250. DOI: 10.1016/j.tibtech.2011.01.007

[125] Matthew MA, Christie J, Yang N, Yao C. A loop-mediated isothermal amplification (LAMP) assay specific to trichomonas tenax is suitable for use at point-of-care. Microorganisms.

Microorganisms. 2022;**10**:594. DOI: 10.3390/microorganisms10030594

[126] Zou Y, Mason MG, Botella JR. Evaluation and improvement of isothermal amplification methods for point-of-need plant disease diagnostics. PLoS One. 2020;**15**(6): e0235216. DOI: 10.1371/journal.pone.0235216

[127] Buscher P, Deborggraeve S. How can molecular diagnostics contribute to the elimination of human African trypanosomiasis? Expert Review of Molecular Diagnostics. 2015;**15**(5): 607-615. DOI: 10.1586/14737159.2015.1027195

[128] Wastling SL et al. LAMP for human African trypanosomiasis: A comparative study of detection formats. PLoS Neglected Tropical Diseases. 2010;**4**(11): e865. DOI: 10.1371/journal.pntd.0000865

[129] Njiru ZK. Rapid and sensitive detection of human African trypanosomiasis by loop-mediated isothermal amplification combined with a lateral-flow dipstick. Diagnostic Microbiology and Infectious Disease. 2011;**69**(2):205-209. DOI: 10.1016/j.diagmicrobio.2010.08.026

[130] Tanner NA, Zhang Y, Evans TC Jr. Visual detection of isothermal nucleic acid amplification using pH-sensitive dyes. BioTechniques. 2015;**58**(2):59-68. DOI: 10.2144/000114253

[131] Pinto J et al. Structural basis for the high specificity of a Trypanosoma congolense immunoassay targeting glycosomal aldolase. PLoS Neglected Tropical Diseases. 2017;**11**(9):e0005932. DOI: 10.1371/journal.pntd.0005932

[132] Pardon E et al. A general protocol for the generation of nanobodies for structural biology. Nature Protocols. 2014;**9**(3):674-693. DOI: 10.1038/nprot.2014.039

[133] Luka G et al. Microfluidics integrated biosensors: A leading technology towards lab-on-a-Chip and Sensing applications. Sensors (Basel). 2015;**15**(12):30011-30031. DOI: 10.3390/s151229783

[134] Hagihara Y, Saerens D. Engineering disulfide bonds within an antibody. Biochimica et Biophysica Acta. 2014; **1844**(11):2016-2023. DOI: 10.1016/j.bbapap.2014.07.005

[135] Muyldermans S. Nanobodies: Natural single-domain antibodies. Annual Review of Biochemistry. 2013; **82**:775-797. DOI: 10.1146/annurev-biochem-063011-092449

[136] Polonelli L et al. Antibody complementarity-determining regions (CDRs) can display differential antimicrobial, antiviral and antitumor activities. PLoS One. 2008; **3**(6):e2371. DOI: 10.1371/journal.pone.0002371

[137] Charles A, Janeway J, Travers P, Walport M, Shlomchik MJ. The structure of a typical antibody molecule, in Immunobiology: The Immune System in Health and Disease. New York: Garland Science; 2001

[138] Kubala MH et al. Structural and thermodynamic analysis of the GFP:GFP-nanobody complex. Protein Science. 2010;**19**(12):2389-2401. DOI: 10.1002/pro.519

[139] Pagneux Q et al. SARS-CoV-2 detection using a nanobody-functionalized voltammetric device. Communications Medicine. 2022;**2**:56. DOI: 10.1038/s43856-022-00113-8

[140] Heukers R, De Groof TWM, Smit MJ. Nanobodies detecting and modulating GPCRs outside in and inside out. Current Opinion in Cell Biology. 2019;**57**:115-122. DOI: 10.1016/j.ceb.2019.01.003

[141] Jovcevska I, Muyldermans S. The therapeutic potential of nanobodies. BioDrugs. 2020;**34**(1):11-26. DOI: 10.1007/s40259-019-00392-z

[142] Sohier JS et al. Allosteric inhibition of VIM metallo-beta-lactamases by a camelid nanobody. The Biochemical Journal. 2013;**450**(3):477-486. DOI: 10.1042/BJ20121305

[143] Staus DP et al. Regulation of beta2-adrenergic receptor function by conformationally selective single-domain intrabodies. Molecular Pharmacology. 2014;**85**(3):472-481. DOI: 10.1124/mol.113.089516

[144] Vincke C, Muyldermans S. Introduction to heavy chain antibodies and derived nanobodies. Methods in Molecular Biology. 2012;**911**:15-26. DOI: 10.1007/978-1-61779-968-6_2

[145] Kariuki CK, Magez S. Improving the yield of recalcitrant nanobodies(R) by simple modifications to the standard protocol. Protein Expression and Purification. 2021;**185**:105906. DOI: 10.1016/j.pep.2021.105906

[146] Scully M et al. Caplacizumab treatment for acquired thrombotic thrombocytopenic purpura. The New England Journal of Medicine. 2019; **380**(4):335-346. DOI: 10.1056/NEJMoa1806311

[147] Kratz F, Elsadek B. Clinical impact of serum proteins on drug delivery. Journal of Controlled Release. 2012; **161**(2):429-445. DOI: 10.1016/j.jconrel.2011.11.028

[148] Wagner TR et al. Neutrobody Plex-monitoring SARS-CoV-2 neutralizing immune responses using nanobodies. EMBO Reports. 2021; **22**(5):e52325. DOI: 10.15252/embr.2020 52325

[149] Li Z et al. An unbiased immunization strategy results in the identification of enolase as a potential marker for nanobody-based detection of Trypanosoma evansi. Vaccines (Basel). 2020;**8**(3):415. DOI: 10.3390/vaccines8030415

[150] Obishakin E et al. Generation of a nanobody targeting the paraflagellar rod protein of trypanosomes. PLoS One. 2014;**9**(12):e115893. DOI: 10.1371/journal.pone.0115893

[151] Ditlev SB et al. Utilizing nanobody technology to target non-immunodominant domains of VAR2CSA. PLoS One. 2014;**9**(1):e84981. DOI: 10.1371/journal.pone.0084981

[152] Deckers N et al. Nanobodies, a promising tool for species-specific diagnosis of taenia solium cysticercosis. International Journal for Parasitology. 2009;**39**(5):625-633. DOI: 10.1016/j.ijpara.2008.10.012

[153] Liu Y et al. Ultrasensitive and highly specific lateral flow assays for point-of-care diagnosis. ACS Nano. 2021;**15**(3): 3593-3611. DOI: 10.1021/acsnano.0c10035

[154] Sena-Torralba A et al. Toward next generation lateral flow assays: Integration of nanomaterials. Chemical Reviews. 2022;**122**(18): 14881-14910. DOI: 10.1021/acs.chemrev.1c01012

[155] Sun W et al. A novel multi-walled carbon nanotube-based antibody

conjugate for quantitative and semi-quantitative lateral flow assays. Bioscience, Biotechnology, and Biochemistry. 2017;**81**(10): 1874-1882. DOI: 10.1080/09168451.2017.1365590

[156] Porras JC et al. Comparative study of gold and carbon nanoparticles in nucleic acid lateral flow assay. Nanomaterials (Basel). 2021;**11**(3):741. DOI: 10.3390/nano11030741

[157] Miller BS et al. Spin-enhanced nanodiamond biosensing for ultrasensitive diagnostics. Nature. 2020; **587**(7835):588-593. DOI: 10.1038/s41586-020-2917-1

[158] Amadeo Sena-Torralba HT-M, Parolo C, Ranjbar S, Nejad MAF, Álvarez-Diduk R, Idili A, et al. A novel Ratiometric fluorescent approach for the modulation of the dynamic range of lateral flow immunoassays. Advanced Materials Technologies. 2022;**7**. DOI: 10.1002/admt.202101450

[159] Shah KG, Yager P. Wavelengths and lifetimes of paper autofluorescence: A simple substrate screening process to enhance the sensitivity of fluorescence-based assays in paper. Analytical Chemistry. 2017;**89**(22):12023-12029. DOI: 10.1021/acs.analchem.7b02424

[160] Dutta Chowdhury A et al. Femtomolar detection of dengue virus DNA with serotype identification ability. Analytical Chemistry. 2018;**90**(21): 12464-12474. DOI: 10.1021/acs.analchem.8b01802

[161] Hajian R et al. Detection of unamplified target genes via CRISPR-Cas9 immobilized on a graphene field-effect transistor. Nature Biomedical Engineering. 2019;**3**(6):427-437. DOI: 10.1038/s41551-019-0371-x

[162] Guo K et al. Rapid single-molecule detection of COVID-19 and MERS antigens via nanobody-functionalized organic electrochemical transistors. Nature Biomedical Engineering. 2021; **5**(7):666-677. DOI: 10.1038/s41551-021-00734-9

[163] Nuzaihan MNM et al. Electrical detection of dengue virus (DENV) DNA oligomer using silicon nanowire biosensor with novel molecular gate control. Biosensors & Bioelectronics. 2016;**83**:106-114. DOI: 10.1016/j.bios.2016.04.033

[164] Dalila RN, Azman MF, Rajaahmoorthi M, Arshad MKM, Fathil MFM, Nuzaihan M, et al. Silicon-on-insulator FET biosensor for dengue DNA complementation. AIP Conference Proceedings. 2018;**2045**(1):020037-7. DOI: 10.1063/1.5080850

[165] Rodriguez MO et al. Silver and gold enhancement methods for lateral flow immunoassays. Talanta. 2016;**148**: 272-278. DOI: 10.1016/j.talanta.2015.10.068

[166] Gao Z et al. Platinum-decorated gold nanoparticles with dual functionalities for ultrasensitive colorimetric in vitro diagnostics. Nano Letters. 2017;**17**(9):5572-5579. DOI: 10.1021/acs.nanolett.7b02385

[167] Arshavsky-Graham S, Segal E. Lab-on-a-chip devices for point-of-care medical diagnostics. Advances in Biochemical Engineering/Biotechnology. 2022;**179**:247-265. DOI: 10.1007/10_2020_127

[168] Lakhin AV, Tarantul VZ, Gening LV. Aptamers: Problems, solutions and prospects. Acta Naturae. 2013;**5**(4):34-43. DOI: 10.32607/20758251-2013-5-4-34-43

[169] Byun J. Recent progress and opportunities for nucleic acid aptamers. Life (Basel). 2021;**11**(3):193. DOI: 10.3390/life11030193

[170] Deroco PB, Kubota DWJLT. Recent advances in point-of-care biosensors for the diagnosis of neglected tropical diseases. Sensors and Actuators B: Chemical. 2021;**349**:130821. DOI: 10.1016/j.snb.2021.130821

[171] Sereno D et al. Isothermal nucleic acid amplification to detect infection caused by parasites of the Trypanosomatidae family: A literature review and opinion on the laboratory to field applicability. International Journal of Molecular Sciences. 2022;**23**(14):7543. DOI: 10.3390/ijms231 47543

[172] Chen JS et al. CRISPR-Cas12a target binding unleashes indiscriminate single-stranded DNase activity. Science. 2018; **360**(6387):436-439. DOI: 10.1126/ science.aar 6245

[173] Li L et al. HOLMESv2: A CRISPR-Cas12b-assisted platform for nucleic acid detection and DNA methylation quantitation. ACS Synthetic Biology. 2019;**8**(10):2228-2237. DOI: 10.1021/ acssynbio.9b00209

[174] Gootenberg JS et al. Multiplexed and portable nucleic acid detection platform with Cas13, Cas12a, and Csm6. Science. 2018; **360**(6387):439-444. DOI: 10.1126/ science.aaq0179

[175] Lee RA et al. Ultrasensitive CRISPR-based diagnostic for field-applicable detection of Plasmodium species in symptomatic and asymptomatic malaria. Proceedings of the National Academy of Sciences of the United States of America. 2020;**117**(41):25722-25731. DOI: 10.1073/ pnas.2010196117

[176] Portney LG, Watkins MP. Foundations of Clinical Research: Applications to Practice. 3rd ed. Philadelphia: F. A. Davis Company; 2015. p. 892. ISBN 10987654321